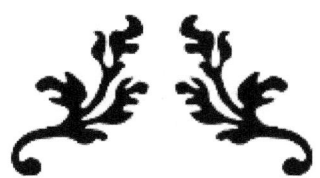

BREAD BAKING FOR BEGINNERS

Sourdough Bread Baking: Keto Bread And Pasta

Mary Nabors

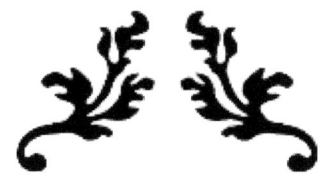

KETO BREAD AND PASTA

Homemade Gluten-Free And Low-Carbohydrate
Baked, Goods For A Healthy Lifestyle, Delicious
Keto Bread And Pasta Recipies To Improve
Weight Loss And Bust Energy

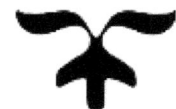

Mary Nabors

Disclaimer

All erudition supplied in this book is specified for educational and academic purposes only. The author is not in any way in charge of any outcomes that emerge from utilizing this book. Constructive efforts have been made to render information that is both precise and effective; however, the author is not to be held answerable for the accuracy or use/misuse of this information.

Foreword

I will like to thank you for taking the very first step of trusting me and deciding to purchase/read this life-transforming book. Thanks for investing your time and resources on this product.

I can assure you of precise outcomes if you will diligently follow the specific blueprint I lay bare in the information handbook you are currently checking out. It has transformed lives, and I firmly believe it will equally change your own life too.

All the information I provided in this Do It Yourself piece is easy to absorb and practice.

Table of Contents

BREAD BAKING BOOK 2

INTRODUCTION

The abundance of bread is one of the leading causes of the current obesity epidemic in westernized societies, but the bread itself is not the cause of the problem. It's what we're using to make the bread that's the primary issue.

Bread is often made with highly processed carb-dense ingredients and served with other calorie-rich foods that are far from healthy for us, but it doesn't have to be that way. Additionally, we can use low-carb flours and other healthy ingredients to make keto-friendly bread and bread products that improve our health and make us feel fuller longer so that we can eat less and feel better than before.

That's why we put together this book with the best recipes for keto bread. With these low-carb bread recipes, you'll be able to satisfy your craving for bread while helping you meet your health and weight loss goals at the same time.

Are you searching for the very best keto pasta for pure nutrition and also wellness from a choice that is also a feasible nutritional perspective that you probably haven't listened to before. The information consisted within this book shares the fact regarding the vital role of a low-carbohydrate, average healthy protein, fat diet plan, in other words, a ketogenic pasta diet regimen can play in improving your overall health and turning around the ill effects of numerous medical conditions as well as chronic diseases. Whatever challenges you encounter as resistance for picking what to consume in this manner, let this book be a reassuring resource of inspiration and also suggestions on your trip to far better health.

This book's aim is mainly to provide you with the knowledge with which to allow the ketogenic diet to run even more smoothly and flawlessly in your everyday life.

UNDERSTANDING KETOSIS

We can refer to ketosis as a metabolic process by which the body does not have sufficient glucose for power. It burns saved fats instead; this leads to an accumulation of acids called ketones within the body. Some individuals encourage ketosis by adhering to a diet called the ketogenic or low-carb diet. The diet plan aims to try and burn unwanted fat forcibly the body to rely on fat for power, instead of carbs.

How do Keto Foods work?

Ketosis is likewise generally observed in individuals with diabetic issues, as the process can occur if the body does not have adequate insulin or is not making use of insulin correctly. Ketosis describes a condition where fat stores are broken down to produce energy, which also generates ketones, a sort of acid. As ketone degrees increase, the acidity of the blood likewise enhances, bringing about ketoacidosis, a severe condition that can confirm fatally.

Some people adhere to a ketogenic (low-carb) diet plan to attempt to slim down by forcing the body to burn fat stores.

In normal circumstances, the body's cells make use of glucose as their primary type of power. The body breaks these down into natural sugars. Sugar can either be used to fuel the body or be stored in the liver as well as muscle mass as glycogen. When the available glucose can't satisfy the power needs, the body will undoubtedly adopt a different approach to meet those requirements. Notably, the body starts to break down fat stored to offer sugar from triglycerides. Ketones are a byproduct of this process; they are acids that do develop in the blood and removed in the urine. In percentages, they serve to suggest that the body is breaking down fat, yet high levels of ketones can toxin the body, causing a procedure called ketoacidosis. Ketosis defines the metabolic state whereby the body transforms fat stores into power, launching ketones while doing so.

The ketogenic diet regimen

As a result of the fact that ketosis breaks down fat stored within the body, some diet regimens intend to produce this metabolic state to facilitate weight-loss.

Ketosis diet plans are also referred to as ketogenic diet plans.

The keto diet plan is typically high in fat. For example, 20% relied on the resource of the calories may be healthy protein, 10% might be carbs, and also 70% might originate from fat. Nevertheless, there are differences, and also the percentages will undoubtedly rely on the variation of the diet plan an individual complies with.

The ketogenic diet plan was additionally used as a treatment for some ailments, although the system for its effectiveness has yet to be revealed. The general public has not been correctly exposed to the truth about ketosis because of some purposeful factors regarding the nutritional adjustments that are needed to induce it. Ketones themselves are generated when the body burns fat, and they're mostly utilized as an alternative fuel source when glucose isn't available.

In other words, your body adjustments from a sugar burner to a fat-burner. Depending on your existing diet regimen and way of life options, becoming keto-adapted can take just a few days and or as long as several weeks or even months. So "staying in ketosis" simply indicates that you are shedding fat. Persistence should be followed to pursue your ketosis.

Is Ketosis Healthy?
The ketogenic diet plan might have a substantial impact on severe wellness conditions, such as:

- heart disease
- diabetic issues
- metabolic disorder

It may additionally boost degrees of HDL cholesterol (high-density lipoproteins, additionally called "good" cholesterol) better than other moderate carbohydrate diets.

These health and wellness advantages could be as a result of the loss of excess weight and also consuming much healthier foods, instead of a decrease in carbohydrates.

The ketogenic diet has likewise been utilized under medical supervision to reduce seizures in kids with epilepsy who do not react to various other types of therapy. Some research studies have recommended that the diet regimen might likewise help adults with epilepsy, although more research study is needed to confirm these searching for.

Various other conditions are likewise being examined to see if a ketogenic diet might be useful; these consist Of:

- Metabolic Syndrome
- Alzheimer's Illness
- Acne
- Cancer Cells
- Polycystic Ovary Illness (Pcos).
- Lou Gehrig's Illness.

BENEFITS OF LOW CARB DIET

For some, they believe that low-carb strategies are efficient in controlling cholesterol levels in the body. This is true that diets short on carbs permit a drop in triglycerides, a body fat-that does not only decrease fat in the body but likewise reduces the possibilities of developing stroke or cardiovascular disease. Another advantage of a diet plan that has very little carb material is that the HDL or the "excellent cholesterol" tends to increase under this condition, which is an advantage.

In regards to LDL or the bad cholesterol, nevertheless, studies have shown that this kind of routine can likewise become crucial in reducing the LDL level as well as in increasing the particle size of the cholesterol, including factor on the part of the diet.

With this evidence at hand, it looks like low-carb plans in basic are winning the battle for being the most satisfactory plan to control cholesterol.

Now, if you want to have more energy, be healthier, look younger, slim down, and cleanse your body, right?

You want to make sure there are plenty of favorable advantages beyond losing weight when you choose a diet plan. You desire to be much healthier overall by consuming in the way the diet plan advises you to consume daily. You likewise wish to have the ability to follow the strategy for life instead of merely a couple of weeks or months. The advantages of a low carbohydrate diet will provide a healthy everyday plan you can implement for life.

You may not understand that consuming carbohydrates can increase the opportunity for adverse health problems. By decreasing the volume of carbohydrates daily of what you eat, some medical conditions you typically experience may occur less naturally.

The frequency of headaches, joint discomfort, and trouble concentrating will reduce when you minimize the intake of carbohydrates. When the pain of joints and problems go away, this might help you reduce the amount of discomfort medicine you take. You will feel much healthier and save more money on medication by the benefits of this diet plan.

Another advantage of the low carb diet is the balancing of state of mind and energy. The body gets more consistent power from protein and other nutrients than from carbohydrates. Carbohydrates bring on short-term energy spurts that will drop your energy level quickly as soon as the carbs are digested. By lowering the volume of carbohydrates you consume, your energy will come from other nutrients that are more consistent energy, decreasing mood, and energy swings.

If you take pleasure in a workout and wish to tone and build muscle tissue that assists fight fat in your body, a low carb diet plan can help. After a workout, your muscles are incredibly delicate to insulin and do not require lots of carbs, as some people might think. By consuming a low carb diet, your muscles after a workout will draw in more amino acids from your meal. The amino acids will assist the muscles to recover from the workout quicker and burn more fat.

A low carbohydrate diet plan can help the effect or avoidance of diabetes. If you have diabetes, a low carb diet may assist in balancing your insulin level more throughout the day. A low carbohydrate diet is an excellent healthy method to stabilize your insulin naturally if you have household members with diabetes and desire to avoid getting the disease yourself.

So as you can see, there are numerous advantages to a low carb diet plan beyond only slimming down. You will see an enhancement in your weight, but you will also have more energy and feel healthier. That is the objective of slimming down as well; to be much healthier.

Eating more vegetables and proteins as well as fruits and nuts can be an excellent way to start a low carb diet. Slowly lower your intake of sweets and foods made from white flour and white sugar. You can discover lots of low carb diet recipes in section two of this book.

Below is the summary of why you should consider a low carb diet?

- Higher HDL Cholesterol.

HDL (high-density lipoprotein) is called the "excellent" cholesterol, and LDL (low-density lipoprotein) is known as the "bad" cholesterol. Current studies have revealed that low carbohydrate diets decrease LDL, and a reduction in bad cholesterol, they also saw a boost in good cholesterol. Excellent cholesterol runs through your bloodstream and, in fact, assists in getting rid of LDL. As HDL gets rid of LDL, it is cleaning your blood system lessening your opportunities for heart problems and stroke.

- Weight Management.

As you will find, eating low carbohydrate is the ideal diet if you have tried to reduce weight and failed in the past. It is effortless to adopt for both weight loss and weight management since it offers so many yummy options. There is a combination of elements that contribute to the effectiveness of the kind of diet plan; Protein permits you to burn energy as opposed to save fat.

- Nutrition.

The low carb diet plan likewise uses a well-balanced diet. Eating fresh meat, fish, veggies, and dairy give you not just healthy choices, but reasonable portions and a variety of foods and meals that keep you satisfied as they are careful to consume. The key is to consume less bad carbs and more good protein combined with high carbs, which consist of low glycemic fresh fruits, like apricots, strawberries, blackberries, and raspberries.

- Lower blood insulin level.

Insulin is a hormonal agent your body uses to store fat. The more bad carbohydrates you eat, the higher your blood insulin level. Consuming low carbohydrate lower your insulin levels by eliminating bad carbohydrates consisting of:

- Fine-tuned grains (white bread, white rice, and enriched pasta).
- Cake, candy cookies, and chips.
- Spud.
- Sweetened sodas.

- Improved Triglycerides.

Triglycerides are storage fats that take a trip in your bloodstream—low carb diets lower triglycerides with the use of meats, green leafy vegetables, and small-carb fruits.

- Minimize Blood Glucose for Diabetics.

Because eating fewer carbohydrates reduces your insulin levels, you are better geared up to keep your blood sugar levels under control, which is a crucial element if you have diabetes.

As you can see, there are numerous rewards to begin a low carbohydrate diet plan and set yourself on the course for a healthier lifestyle. Stay alive and live healthily.

WHY YOU SHOULD INCREASE YOUR PROTEIN INTAKE

How much protein do you need for a healthy life? Proteins have vital roles in all aspects of your body's function; it is count among the essential nutrient elements of your diet plan. Striking the ideal protein content in your daily diet can do great things to your general health.

The question is, how much is the right quantity?

There is plenty of details from a range of sources concerning the correct amount of proteins. However, the reality is that none of these sources knows you. If there is anyone qualified to choose your maximum protein requirements, it is you; because dietary protein requirements are governed by aspects like body weight and exercise, which only you will completely understand.

How Much Protein?

There is a lot of research data offered relating to the correct amount of protein for an adult. And, there is a considerable quantity of variation in the guidelines that each research result supplies. However, something that a majority of results appears to agree upon is the range of 0.6-0.8 grams of protein per kilo of body weight or 0.27-0.36 grams per pound of body weight. The majority of research study results seem to point towards the higher limitation;

therefore, you can safely determine your protein requirements at 0.36 grams per pound of body weight. That exercises to around 54 grams of protein a day for an adult weighing 150 pounds. Now, whether your body weight is ideal is something you will need to discover on the Body Mass Index (BMI) scale, which you will certainly learn about.

Where do I get my proteins?

If you are an adult with a standard 9 to 5 routine, your protein requirements will be immediately looked after in your regular diet. This is assuming the reality that your daily diet is a healthy mix of whole grain, bread, eggs, milk, meat, and veggies. You are taking care of your body's protein requirement if the presumption is right. Everything you consume, ranging from bread to baked beans, contributes towards your protein consumption, and hitting the minimum protein requirement will be an easy job for anybody who does not avoid meals.

If you wish to know the exact amount of protein you get from various sources just to be sure, then here are the details. Eggs, milk, and meat are the most significant factors. An egg offers you 6.5 grams, while 100 grams of chicken gives you 26 grams, and a cup of skimmed milk contributes around 8.35 grams. It is the vegetarians who need to be slightly more conscious about their protein consumption as vegetables are not especially rich in proteins. In such cases, consuming the correct amount of cereals and complementing them with foodstuffs like almonds can settle the concern.

Why can't I just store?

There is a misunderstanding that just excess of fats and carbohydrates are bad for health; which an excess consumption of protein can refrain from doing much harm. This is incorrect. Excess use of proteins is a concern on the kidneys and the general metabolism. Protein intake does not directly transform into muscle mass, and excess proteins are, in some cases, metabolically converted to fat. So, grabbing all of the proteins is not a good concept at all.

I exercise, should I consume more?

Research has shown that there is no excessive link between protein intake and athletic efficiency, and more surprisingly, these findings even obtain weight trainers. You require to increase your protein intake if you work out frequently dynamically. The suggestions lie at 1-1.2 grams per kg of body weight for expert athletes. Presuming you are not a professional, a new glass of milk may just serve.

So you wish to slim down or include muscle. That sounds near basically everyone's goals. One crucial element in identifying whether you'll have success in this endeavor is your protein consumption and general nutritional options. A high protein diet results in a favorable nitrogen state, which potentiates muscle development.

A high protein diet plan is shown to be thermogenic, which leads to increased calorie burning and, consequently, increased weight loss. A high protein diet plan has likewise been revealed to increase the release of the hormone glucagon. Glucagon is a hormone that is understood to help avoid fat storage.

No matter how far one desire to change their body, a high protein diet plan will be required to achieve any real success.

WHAT IS GLUTEN

You might have asked if gluten-free is the way to go if you also heard of the incredible health benefits. Knowing how to recognize it and avoid it is vital to your health. What is gluten?

Gluten is a group of proteins found in many grains such as wheat, barley, or rye. Gluten makes dough sticky and causes bread to be fluffy and airy. Gluten is considered a "sticky" protein since it holds together nutrition storage areas in plants. Gluten is frequently utilized by food producers as a binder and filler. Gluten binds to the lining of the little intestinal tract, triggering significant swelling as your body attacks the cells of your small intestinal tract. Agonizing inflammation also occurs, making you unable to absorb the nutrients you consume from food. Too much exposure to gluten can result in a dripping gut. Celiac illness is the most severe condition associated with gluten. Those who have been detected with celiac need to follow a gluten-free diet prepare for a lifetime. To determine and prevent gluten, you need to read the ingredients labels. There are familiar sources of gluten, but you should be mindful of concealed sources of this toxic protein.

It is a composite of 4 kinds of proteins: prolamins, albumins, globulins, and glutelins. These are plant storage proteins. Albumin and globulins prevail in may grains, including grains acceptable on a gluten-free diet plan, such as corn and rice.

When it comes to gluten intolerance, prolamins and glutenins are the real perpetrators. They exist in the cereal grains or grassy grains connected to wheat, such as barley, rye, spelled Kamut, and triticale. In these grains, the glutelins and prolamins comprise as much as eighty percent of the protein composite that constitutes gluten.

What Foods Contain Gluten?

Seasonings such as curries, sauces such as soy sauce, and barbecue sauce often hide the sources of gluten in them. Supplements and vitamins, in some cases, have gluten in them as a binder or filler. Taste enhancer ingredients such as hydrolyzed protein or autolyzed yeast extract may have this damaging protein composite in them.

Typical Gluten Food Sources:

- Any Kind Of Rye, Barley Or Wheat:
- Bread
- Cakes
- Cereals
- Cookies
- Crackers
- Muffins
- Pancakes
- Pasta
- Pies
- Pretzels
- Waffles

Gluten in not-so-obvious food sources:

- Alcohol.
- Candy.

- Cold Cuts And Luncheon Meats.
- Corn Chips.
- Dry Roasted Nuts.
- Gravy Cubes.
- Chicken, Meat, And Vegetable Stock Cubs.
- Processed Crab.

What is Gluten-Free and Leading a Non-Gluten Life.

Gluten-free is a kind of diet that is devoid of food containing gluten. To recognize what is gluten-free, you should initially understand gluten is. Leading a non-gluten life is necessary for people who have celiac illness, gluten intolerance, dermatitis herpetiformis, wheat allergy, and migraines. If gluten-containing foods are taken in, individuals with sensitivity to gluten might experience signs comparable to those for irritable bowel syndrome. Some of these signs consist of diarrhea, constipation, bloating, gas, weakness, and so on. People who have high sensitivity to gluten are advised to eliminate it from their diet or to reduce its consumption to avoid this problem.

What Is Gluten Intolerance?

Some people who take gluten develop allergic reactions or intolerances. As a result of studies, it has been discovered that in America, about one in ten people develop a certain degree of sensitivity to gluten. It has just recently been approximated that nearly one in ten individuals in the United States experience some degree of a level of sensitivity to gluten.

The most severe kind of gluten intolerance is celiac disease. When someone struggles with gluten intolerance, antibodies assault the lining of his or her little intestinal tract, causing swelling and slowly exterminating the microvilli along the digestive wall. This makes it so that toxic substances can more easily enter the bloodstream through the gastrointestinal wall and makes it more difficult for the individual to absorb their food to obtain essential nutrients correctly.

What Are Gluten Intolerance Symptoms?

The most typical gluten intolerance signs are gastrointestinal. These symptoms include flatulence, cramping, bloating, and rotating cases of diarrhea and irregularity. The malnutrition that results from using down the microvilli and irritating the small intestinal tract's lining may produce a variety of signs related to malnutrition that can be tough to mention. This is one reason gluten intolerance is so frequently misdiagnosed or missed entirely. The majority of gluten intolerant people respond well to a gluten-free diet; however, you desire to ensure this really is your disorder before you try to remove such a typical staple in the American diet.

In the market place, more flour choices than ever before are available to accommodate the gluten-free diet, such include:

- Brown Rice Flour.

This is an extra flour and works excellent when mixed with teff, sorghum or buckwheat flours. It is excellent for cooking and works for both mouthwatering and sweet meals.

- Millet Flour.

This is a light in color and drier flour than others are and is best when blended with heartier flours, like, Teff, Hemp, or almond, but it should not be utilized by itself.

- Teff Flour.

Teff is a well-rounded flour that works terrific for baking in gluten-totally free diet plans. It is loaded with high nutrients and has a nutty flavor and darker color. This flour is not easily found in standard markets but can be gotten online.

- Buckwheat Flour.

This is a perfect gluten complimentary flour option for usage in cakes, muffins, and pancakes. Buckwheat pancakes are much healthier as far as weight management than the standard white flour ranges. In order to get a dough that rolls well, include something starchy, such as cornstarch or tapioca flour.

- Sweet White Rice Flour (Mochiko).

This is an excellent choice to add wetness and density to baked goods. It has a slightly milky taste, and it's a little sweet. It is usually used to make Japanese desserts such as Mochi. It works well for both mouthwatering and delicious dishes.

- Almond Flour.

This is an excellent choice for baking. Made from ground almonds, it is also a fantastic choice for shallow carb baking. Utilizing 1/4 of this in any flour mixture will add moistness, binding, a light almond taste, and a right amount of density to muffins, brownies, cookies, bread, dehydrated snacks, and cake recipes.

- Corn Flour.

Corn flour can be contributed to numerous gluten-free flour blends, flatbreads, and pasta.

Benefits Of Gluten-Free Diet

In today's world, many individuals are choosing to go gluten-free. For some, it is because of a current medical diagnosis, and for others, it is because of the recent promotion about the favorable health advantages a gluten-free diet plan provides.

Celiac disease is not the only reason that individuals all over the world are changing their eating routines to adjust to a gluten-free diet. There are numerous other health benefits to this diet plan that will help anyone with or without celiac illness. For individuals without the disease, they have the advantage of not needing to make extreme modifications to their lifestyle to delight in the health advantages such as weight-loss. They can make some small changes to the particular components they put in their food and be a much healthier person and, of course, slim down.

The quantity of calcium your body absorbs will increase daily. This is very important for the health of your bones, teeth, and muscle contractions. Your bones will become more powerful, and their density will likewise be enhanced.

For kids and infants who are looking to gain from this in more ways than just their more powerful bones and immune system, there is much less opportunity of them developing asthma or allergic reactions at an early age when following this diet.

Your bloodstream will have lower levels of triglyceride. If you do not know what triglyceride is, it is a mix of three fatty acids, and high levels of it have been connected to heart disease, hardening of the arteries, and stroke. The gluten-free diet has been proven to make people's bodies feel excellent and feel much healthier, and a healthy person is a delighted person.

Here are some of the claims that have actually been made about the benefits of excluding gluten from one's diet plan:

1. Faster recovery time

For weightlifters and professional athletes, this is one of the most frequently pointed out advantages of a gluten-free diet. A gluten-free diet plan might have a definite edge on decreasing one's healing time after exercise. It's somewhat arguable whether or not a gluten-free diet will shorten the healing time for everybody. However, it definitely can certainly offer benefits for those people who have a gluten-intolerance. Today, there are increasingly more "recovery" beverages and foods on the marketplace that are gluten-free.

2. Enhanced gut motility and function

Scientific research studies show that those people with gluten intolerance are more susceptible to having numerous digestion issues, such as Irritable Bowel Syndrome (IBS). The service is to start a gluten-free diet that doesn't contain individual entire grains.

3. Less Immune System Overload

When your body's intake of iron is too expensive, your immune system fails to operate at an optimum level. Body immune system Overload triggers no signs, so it's vital to have specific blood tests done to identify whether you have it. While there are various effective methods to minimize the quantity of iron that you take in, one approach is to modify your diet plan. That includes beginning and preserving a gluten-free diet.

4. Minimized Systemic Inflammation (SI).

This is among the commonly cited advantages of a gluten complimentary diet plan. While the process of SI is technical and rather intricate, it can result in numerous unwanted conditions that result from a weaker body immune system. To counter the procedure of systemic swelling, specialists suggest that sufferers of SI begin consuming a diet that consists strictly of plant-based foods and whole foods. They also recommend that people with SI likewise consume diets that are devoid of specific compounds, consisting of Casein and Gluten. Such actions can provide an affordable and effective method to identify the causes of one's problems with SI.

5. Enhanced nutrient absorption from food.

A heavily grain-based diet plan appears to produce some unfavorable impacts on the body's capability to soak up nutrients from food. For instance, a diet high in gluten can cause celiac illness, which can harm things called villi, which are included in a person's digestive lining.

WHAT IS KETO PASTA

While different kinds of pasta are loaded with carbohydrates and as a result not keto-friendly, there are ways one can enjoy a pasta even on a keto diet. Among the most convenient methods to shift to a keto diet is to find a low-carb replacement for your favorite foods rather than banning them entirely from your diet. That's right-- you can have noodles on a low-carb diet plan. Pasta is a staple in almost every cooking area, so it's no wonder they have their very own aisle in the supermarket.

However, these delicious pasta dishes are good news for your health level and also ketone degrees. This overview will certainly help you understand why most pasta is fit for a keto diet plan as well as how you can locate enjoyable options to help you stay on track with your wellness objectives.

What Are Pasta and Why Aren't They Low-Carb or Keto-Friendly?

The first record of pasta dates back to 4,000 years back in China, although these high-carb strips have spread throughout the world. Keto pasta is a critical component in the standard meals of numerous cultures around the world, such as the Italians as well as Eastern cuisines. Pasta is made from a flour-and-egg dough, which is extended and also rolled flat before being cut into long, slices. Often made from wheat flour, they are categorized as a grain product, they are usually made with unleavened dough, which implies there was no chemical or artificial leavening contributed to making the mixture surge.

Regarding the preparation, noodles can be boiled, tossed in a mix fry, or deep-fried. Traditional noodle recipes usually are eaten with eggs or with some kind of sauce or soup.

One cup (160 grams) of typically cooked egg noodles contains an overall of 221 calories, including 40 grams of carbs, 38 grams of net carbs, 2 grams of fiber, 3 grams of fat, and also 7 grams of protein.

Low-Carb Substitutes For Pasta

Provided the high quantity of carbohydrates in one cup of regular pasta, it's not a surprise they aren't low-carb or keto-friendly. But that doesn't mean you can't still enjoy your pasta as a keto meal.

There are plenty of low-carb noodles as well as pasta choices available today, similar to there is low-carb bread. Several of these fantastic low-carb noodles consist of:

- Shirataki Noodles
- Zoodles
- Low-Carb Egg Noodles
- Pasta Squash

1. Shirataki Noodles

Shirataki noodles, also referred to as wonder noodles, are just one of the leading zero-carb, calorie-free noodles you can safely consume on the ketogenic diet plan. Being the only carb-free noodles out there today, it's no surprise they're called a wonder. This noodle type is own by the Japanese extracted from a yam type called "Konjac" Not just are they vegan as well as low-carb friendly, they're essentially unsavory too. They absorb the flavor as well as shade of whatever they're prepared with.

Unlike a lot of noodles and pasta today, shirataki noodles are most typically pre-packaged in liquid. The fluid tends to have a shady odor, which leads some to think the noodles have to taste in this manner. Just bring out your bowl-shaped sieve and give them a thorough rinsing in the cold, running water, and the odor disappears totally.

Around 97% of shirataki noodle content is water, as well as the various other 3% is a water-soluble fiber called glucomannan. This incredible noodle has no calories. One offering size (three ounces) additionally has 0 grams of fat, less than 1 gram of carbohydrates, and 0 grams of healthy protein.

Toss these simple konjac noodles with a little sesame oil, keto chicken or shrimp, coconut oil instead of soy sauce, add all the veggies you love, and you can still stir fry it.

Luckily, shirataki noodles can be discovered in a lot of food stores today. Provide a shot as well as begin giving your favorite noodle-based dishes a low-carb spin.

2. Zoodles

An additional enjoyable way to include noodles to your keto meals without including carbohydrates is zoodles. What are zoodles?

Zoodles or "zucchini noodles" can be discovered pre-packaged in the fruit and vegetable area of your neighborhood supermarket or can be quickly developed in your area.

Zoodles are made by spiralizing your preferred veggies right into ribbon-shaped noodles; it's that simple. While the "z" in zoodles represents zucchini, you can make noodles out of various vegetables, including carrots and beets. Nonetheless, zucchini consists of the most affordable carbohydrate count.

Unlike regular noodles, zoodles are wheat-free, vegan, grain-free, gluten-free, as well as incredibly nutritious. Have a look at the nutrition facts: One cup of zoodles or "zucchini noodles" has 20 grams of calories, including less than 1 gram of fat, 4 grams of carbohydrates, 2.5 grams of net carbs, 1.5 grams of fiber, and also 1.5 grams of healthy protein.

Along with being the perfect low-carb noodle alternative, zoodles also provide plentiful health and wellness advantages. Zoodles are a high source of antioxidants, have anti-inflammatory homes, supply an abundant amount of potassium, aid improve food digestion as well as eye wellness, and also can even help people experiencing diabetes mellitus as well as excessive weight.

3. Low-Carb Egg Noodles

Wish to get creative with your pasta? Attempt making your low-carb egg noodles in the house. It's less complicated than you assume.

4. Spaghetti Squash

Last but not least, another prominent best choice for the whole low-carb pasta or noodle is spaghetti squash. Not only is it low incomplete carbohydrates and also high in fiber, but this big yellow vegetable is also packed with a dietary worth that will keep you invigorated throughout the day.

Accurately how do you correctly prepare spaghetti squash?

To transform your pasta squash into the perfect low- calorie, low-carb noodle alternative, you'll need to comply with a couple of easy actions:

- Preheat the stove to 400 ° F.
- Cut the spaghetti squash in half pieces.
- Drizzle olive oil, salt, and also pepper on the squash.
- Set on a flat pan and bake in the oven for about 40 to 45 minutes.

One cup of spaghetti squash has a total amount of 31 calories that includes less than 1 gram of fat, 7 grams of carbs, 5.5 grams of fiber, 1.5 grams of net carbohydrates, and less than 1 gram of protein.

With the essential nutrients and fiber this vegetable offers, you'll be satisfied without any fear of obtaining tossed out of ketosis.

Try these shirataki pasta keto style and more if you have been really feeling robbed of an excellent low-carb noodle alternative that fits your keto diet, you currently have choices. With these low-carb replacements, there is no limit to the noodle recipes you can make while adhering to a low-carb or ketogenic diet plan.

Do yourself a favor and also attempt any of these noodle choices today. You'll get guilt-free happiness of noodles with all the additional benefits your preferred noodle replacement has to offer.

Options To Prepare Keto Pasta

The good news is, there's no demand to quit your favored pasta dishes, simply use low carb pasta noodles in your preferred recipes.

So, how do you make low carbohydrate pasta? You can re-create the majority of your favorite pasta meals to be keto-friendly, you simply have to make use of small carb noodles.

Simply comply with these simple steps for exactly how to make keto pasta:

- Select the reduced carbohydrate pasta alternative you're going to use. Will you make a homemade reduced carbohydrate pasta? Or pick a store-bought option?
- Some are made out of vegetables, and also others are made from a reduced carb pasta dough.
- Include flavor to your low carbohydrate pasta dish with your favorite keto pasta sauce.
- Offer your low carb pasta with garnishes if appropriate and get your forks ready for pasta twirling!

With a couple of exemptions, most reduced carb pasta replacements are made from vegetables. Naturally, these are not similar to traditional wheat pasta, yet they can still be scrumptious and offer up more nourishment for you.

Necessary Tools To Make Keto Pasta.
If you're making veggie noodles, you'll need a minimum of one of these tools:

- Tabletop Spiralizer-- This handy gizmo makes the best-reduced carb pasta dishes! If you intend to make great deals of spiralized veggies, you'll want the tabletop variation.
- Hand-Held Spiralizer-- This spiralizer is much smaller in size; however, it still functions well and also is perfect if you are cooking for one or two or if you have no cooking area storage for the tabletop version.
- Mandoline Slicer-- The quickest method to slice up veggie in thin parts. Perfect for making low carbohydrate noodles for pasta.

KETO BREAD

There's really no mystery about bread baking, and it's one of the most natural things to do, even though most people may think that bread baking is a tough task. But that is not true. You need just a few things to be in place in other to produce the perfect bread. There are, therefore, only four necessary ingredients to make a loaf of bread: flour, yeast, sugar, and water. In addition, it is required to add salt for the sake of flavor and to keep the yeast from growing too quickly. Keto has helped many people lose weight, the laws of what you can and can't eat are quite limiting.

In general, you can aim to eat less than 50 carbs a day to keep your body in a fat-burning state of ketosis. The average macro breakdown is 70 to 80 percent fat, 15 to 20 percent protein, and 5 to 10 percent carbohydrate.

Studies have noted that while the typical slice of bread is usually around 10 to 20 grams of carbs, you can make bread with other low-carb ingredients such as almond flour, coconut flour, psyllium husk, cream cheese, and eggs. You'll learn more about Keto bread and their recipes in this book. Certain ingredients may be added to make various types of bread. Of starters, if you add butter and eggs, you're going to have Challah or Egg Bread. Some ingredients that can be added are nuts, olives, onions, and molasses instead of sugar or honey.

Some of the types of flour used for bread are All-Purpose Flour or Bread Flour, Whole Wheat Flour, and Rye Flour. Cornmeal may be substituted for some flour, and oats may also be used in baking. Yeast comes in a dry granulated form, and this is the easiest way to make use of it. It can also be bought in a cake shape. Dry yeast is sold on the market in strips of 3 packages. Warehouse type stores also sell 1 lb—packets of yeast. Place your yeast in the refrigerator, and this will increase the shelf life of your yeast. Sweeteners widely used in bread are sugar, honey, molasses, and malt powder, or simply allow the yeast to extract its nutrition from the sugar commonly found in the flour.

Bread is made from flour, i.e., grain, which has been ground into powder. The quality of bread depends to no small extent on the protein content of the flour. Better bread use flour containing 12 to 14 percent protein rather than all-purpose wheat flour containing just 9 to 12 percent protein. Keto bread tastes really eggy and can quickly be fallen apart.

A list of low-carb flours in our Keto kitchen

- Coconut flour
- Almond flour

1. Coconut flour.

Coconut flour food contains few carbohydrates and can be considered keto food. You have seen and heard all the ketogenic benefits of coconut oil; it is everywhere; many of us consume it every day. Another part of the coconut that interests us most today is "coconut flour."

Coconut flour is an ideal substitute for low-carb flour for cakes, brownies, and cupcake dishes when you want a moist consistency. " We use coconut flour in our dishes for keto cooking because of the tiny number of "carbohydrates." Although it is not a carbohydrate-free flour, the coconut flour itself is not moist; It attracts moisture from other components and acquires the consistency of things like eggs and water.

The ability of coconut flour to absorb moisture causes foods like our Keto muffins (listed below) to become moist and smooth without drying out, unlike the other low-carb flours we use, which combine better. With cookies and crusts.

2.   Almond flour.

Another essential component in many of our LCHF baking dishes and desserts is olive flour. Olive flour is just ground almonds, blanched without the skin.

Almond flour is an extremely flexible component to have in the kitchen; We use it in various keto cooking dishes. Almond flour is the main active keto ingredient in our low-carbohydrate carbohydrates.

Equipment Needed In Kitchen
Essential tools that are relevance:

- Bench scraper
- Bowl scraper
- Bread knife
- Cooling rack
- Dutch oven

- Scale - however truly, this one is essential
- Containers or little plastic food storage containers
- Kitchen area towels or cling wrap
- Lame or very sharp blade or knife
- Mixing bowls
- Thermometers
- Oven thermometer
- Probe thermometer
- Ambient temperature level thermometer

These tools are used with less frequency but still appropriate to the house baker's toolbox:

- Banneton basket
- Baking pan
- Baking stone
- Cleaning up brushes
- Cutters
- Flour wand
- Oven bags
- Rolling pin
- Scoop

IMPORTANT OF KETO PASTA AND KETO BREAD

Now you know that the keto pasta diet is a low-sugar, low-carbohydrate technique of eating with the end goal of placing the body into a state of ketosis. When ketosis is accomplished, the body quits relying on sugar for power and also begins melting fat instead. Ketosis can lead to a variety of health benefits, from weight reduction to an increase in brain features.

So if ketosis is your goal, you can explore a massive plate of pasta for supper. One piece of great information, however, is that medical professionals typically advise that individuals do the keto diet regimen in cycles as opposed to adopting it as a way of life. Keto can be a fantastic means to start fat burning, yet it can be hard on the body long- term. In other words, you can have pasta again someday.

Right here are some of the many health and wellness advantages that come from consuming Keto Pasta:

- All-natural appetite control
- Effortless weight loss as well as maintenance
- Mental clarity
- Sounder, a lot more restful sleep
- Stabilized metabolic function

- Stabilized blood glucose and bring back insulin level of sensitivity
- Reduced inflammation degrees
- Sensations of joy and essential wellness
- Lowered high blood pressure
- Increased HDL (good) cholesterol
- Minimized triglycerides
- Decreased or gotten rid of little LDL fragments (harmful cholesterol).
- Capability to go twelve to twenty-four hours between meals.
- Use kept body fat as a gas resource.
- Countless energy.
- Removed heartburn.
- Much better fertility.
- Avoidance of traumatic mind injury.
- It increases sex drive.
- It enhances the body's immune system.
- It reduced aging due to a decrease in totally free extreme production.
- Improvements in blood chemistry.
- Optimized cognitive features and also enhanced memory.
- Minimized acne outbreaks and also other skin problems.
- Increased understanding of just how foods influence your body.
- Improvements in metabolic health pens.
- Faster as well as much better recuperation from exercise.
- Reduced anxiety and mood swings.

I think you understand. Ketosis is something you might wish to pursue if you are taking care of weight or health and wellness concerns, and also you're not getting the outcomes you want with your present method.

In sections two and three of this book, we will certainly review many keto bread and keto pasta dishes that are significantly enhanced by a ketogenic diet regimen, also responding much better to it than to several of the best medications readily available. It's incredible to think that you might see such outstanding development making use of nourishment instead of a drug.

SECTION TWO
RECIPES FOR KETO BREAD

These ketogenic bread recipes will undoubtedly enable you to enjoy various types of bread with low carb. Bread is just one of the most widely eaten foods in westernized cultures. In the United States, it is the second most generally eaten food, following closely behind grain-based treats.

Bread is often made with highly processed carb-dense with active ingredients offered with other calorie-rich foods that form against healthy and balanced for us, yet it doesn't need to be in this manner. Conversely, we can make use of low-carb flours as well as various other healthy ingredients to make keto-friendly bread and also bread items that improve our wellness and even make us feel fuller longer so that we can lastly consume less and look as well as feel better than before. With these low-carb bread dishes, you will certainly have the ability to please your craving for bread while it aids you to satisfy your health and also weight-loss objectives at the same time.

Keto Zucchini Bread

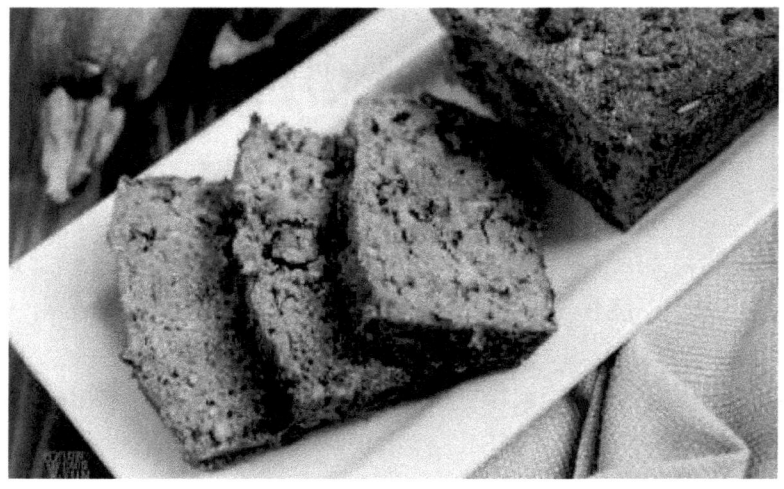

Zucchini is so flexible that it makes fries, zoodles, lasagna, and now you can make zucchini bread that will contribute to your keto bread collection. Many people think that traditional zucchini bread is too sweet, and it's not surprising because the meals require two or more cups of sugar. The truth is that in this zucchini keto recipe with bread, you don't have to overload it with sugar. A small amount of vanilla extract contains the exact amount of sweet flavor for this delicious loaf of bread.

In addition to cutting the sugar, we can use coconut and almond flour instead of soft flour. This method eliminates grains, reduces carbohydrates, and balance the protein.

The health benefits of zucchini

Not only have we removed some of the unhealthy portions that are commonly found in sweetbread, but we also include the health benefits of zucchini. Here are some of its incredible benefits:

- Potassium: This mineral is useful for controlling high blood pressure. The serving size is more than 15% of the recommended daily value.
- Low in calories: Include zucchini into your bread by reducing total calories.
- Gastrointestinal Benefits: The high moisture content of zucchini and other zucchini during the summer season is generally recommended to relieve inflammation in the digestive system.
- It contains a small number of carbohydrates, just a little bit essential for a keto diet.
- Anti-inflammatory agent: help your body heal among miraculous natural foods.

Ingredients

- 4 medium eggs (176 g).
- 1 large zucchini, crushed (pressed moisture) (about 1 to 2 cups).
- Half /2 cup of almond flour (60 g).
- Quarter cup coconut flour (28 g).
- 8 tablespoons of coconut oil (120 ml).
- 1 teaspoon of baking powder (2 g).
- 1 teaspoon of vanilla extract (5 ml).
- A pinch of salt.

Instructions.

- Preheat the oven to 350 F (175 C).
- Combine all the components in a large bowl.
- Make sure to squeeze out all the moisture from the zucchini.
- Pour into a bread pot and bake for 50 minutes.
- Let cool and place.

Keto Almond Bread Recipe

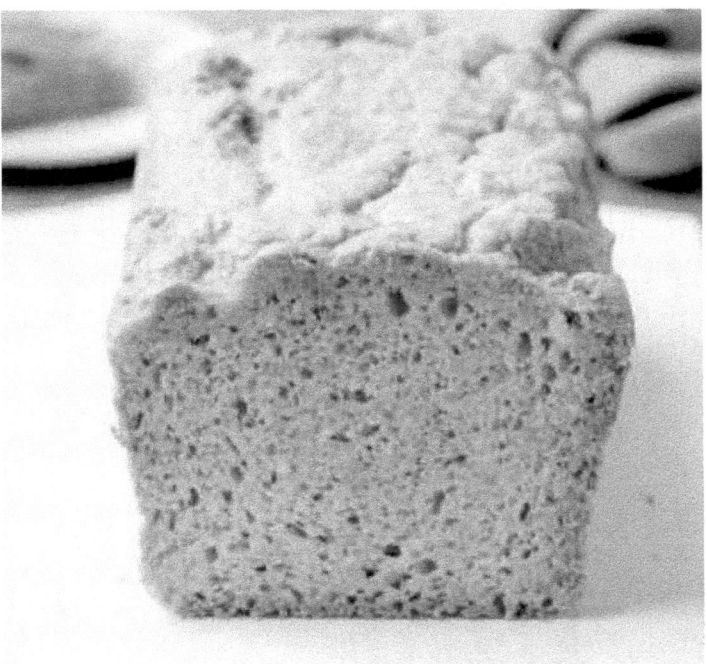

Some of you may be on a keto diet to control your blood sugar. Almond flour is a great way to achieve this goal. Routine bread with refined wheat is not only rich in carbohydrates, but also low in fiber and fat. This combination can cause harmful splashes of blood sugar. This bread keeps carbs under control while increasing fat and fiber, which releases blood sugar more slowly.

Almond flour has many health benefits, such as:

- Gluten free
- Good heart
- Extremely for people with high cholesterol.

- Low in carbohydrates
- Fiber content
- It is rich in protein
- Blood sugar control.

How to use this flour.

It will probably not take you long to integrate bread successfully into your life. I'm sure you already imagine the possibilities, but here are some suggestions:

- Sandwiches
- With a bowl of soup.
- Crunchy bread.
- Regular toasts

Ingredients.

- Two beaten eggs.
- One cup of (120 g) almond flour.
- 1.5 teaspoons of baking powder (3 g).
- 3 tablespoons of olive oil (45 ml).
- 1 teaspoon powdered mustard (2 g) or other herbs/spices of your choice (optional, omit if used to make French toast).
- One teaspoon of coarse salt (5 g) (optional, you can omit).
- 1 teaspoon instant gluten-free yeast in combination with 1 tablespoon (15 ml) lukewarm water (optional).

Instructions.

- Preheat oven to 350 F (180 C).
- Combine eggs, almond flour, baking powder, mustard powder, salt, and olive oil. If you are using an optional yeast mixture (to add "flavor," it is entirely voluntary), add it now.
- Mix well to form a sticky paste.
- Place the mixture on a small greased baking sheet (3.5 inches x 8 inches / 9 cm x 20 cm) and smooth over the top.
- Bake for 30 minutes.
- After baking, carefully tilt and cut into four squares, which is the size of a slice of bread, which essentially results in 4 thick slices (something like focaccia or a hamburger).

Hey, it's okay if your mind is continuously wandering around the bread as soon as you start the Keto lifestyle, but satisfy those thoughts with a great keto-friendly version. Olive flour is a saving grace on this bread plate that keeps it low in carbohydrates, which means you can have your bread and eat it!

Pumpkin Bread

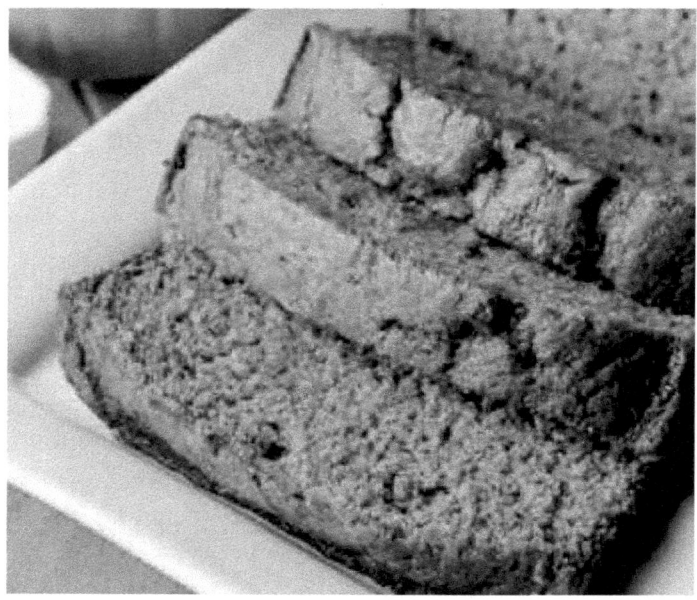

There are ingredients that keep us company not only in fall however also in the first cold winters, such as pumpkin! After using it for numerous preparations, such as tasty lasagna or creamy velvety, we thought of a home-made leavened with love: a soft and aromatic pumpkin bread! Delicate and smooth, with a neutral flavor that goes well with both sweet and mouthwatering, this bread will be the king of your table. Place it in the center, surrounded by meats, jams, and cheeses: everyone can select their own pairing, and fill their own wedge as they choose! Bread enthusiasts, simply like us, will taste it alone, since pumpkin bread is so great that it does not require anything else!

INGREDIENTS

363 CALORIES PER SERVING

- Dry brewer's yeast 4 g.
- 00 flour 500 g.
- Raw tidy pumpkin 400 g.
- Malt 5 g.
- Extra virgin olive oil 20 g.
- Salt approximately 10 g.
- Pumpkin seeds 15 g.
- Room temperature water 100 g.
- 2 sprigs rosemary.

PREPARATION.

- To prepare the pumpkin bread, start by cleaning it: eliminate the seeds and internal filaments and suffice into wedges, and likewise eliminate the peel.
- Place a pan with water on the stove and flavor with rosemary. Place the pumpkin wedges in the steaming basket and cover.
- Cook the pumpkin: it will take about 30 minutes, it needs to be soft and firm, you can inspect its consistency with the prongs of a fork.
- Pass the prepared pulp with a potato masher in order to obtain a puree.
- In a planetary mixer sort, the flour then adds the pumpkin puree, the yeast, and malt.
- Place the hook and operate the planetary mixer at low speed, and include the water flush, it is essential that it is at room temperature level.

- Continue to knead, increasing the speed, for a minimum of 10 minutes. When the dough is stringed, you can include salt: do not add it faster because if inserted too early, it would prevent the dough from increasing.
- Let the salt soak up by continuing to knead for 2 minutes, then add the oil to wire and let it soak up too: it will take about 3 minutes. Transfer the dough to the work surface area, roll it out a little and continue with the folds: fold the side flaps and then the upper and lower ones, as if to make a bundle.
- It is sealed to form a ball and place it to increase in a large bowl. Cover with cling film and let the dough rise for at least 3 hours in a warm location (for instance, the oven switched off with the light on) up until it doubles in volume.
- Gently flour the work surface and put the leavened dough into it. Carry out the four folds of force once again, form a well-sealed ball as previously and position it on the baking tray covered with parchment paper.
- Let rise for another 1 hour then, with a well-sharpened knife or with a cutter, make 8 cuts on the surface area of the dough to make it comparable to a real pumpkin.
- Steam some water on the surface of the bread to make it wet, and disperse the pumpkin seeds inside the grooves you have actually sculpted.
- Bake the bread now in a static oven preheated to 200 °, on the bottom of which you will have put a pan with water, for the very first twenty minutes:

the water will form inside the oven the humidity required for the right leavening.

- After the very first 20 minutes, remove the pan of water, lower the temperature level to 190 ° and cook the bread for another 35 minutes.
- Let your pumpkin bread cool off prior to enjoying it!

STORAGE.

As you know, the bread is good fresh: if possible, consume it throughout the day. You can keep it in a paper bag for about three days. You can also freeze pumpkin bread, entire or currently cut into comfy wedges if you have actually used just fresh and not thawed active ingredients.

Recommendations.

Pumpkin or courgettes? With the dough, you can make a "family size" bread-like ours, or divide it between making small sandwiches. An excellent idea to prepare really original burgers!

Quick Keto Toast

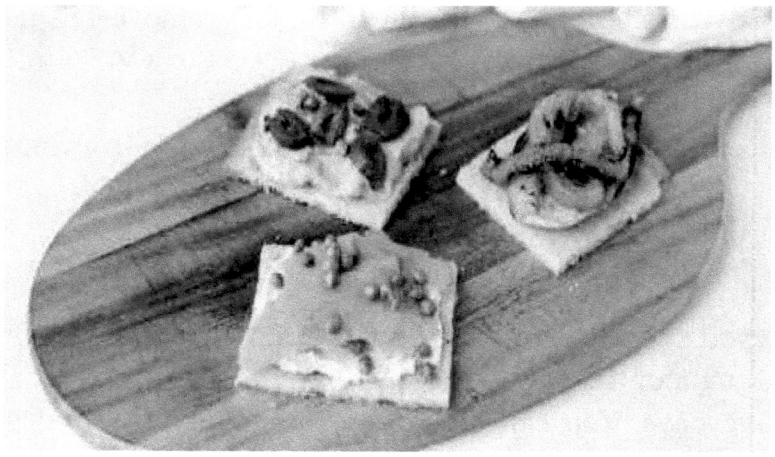

This Keto toast recipe takes a little more effort than sticking pieces of store-bought white bread into a toaster. However, this recipe allows you to consume delicious bread that's Keto, low carb, dairy-free, and Paleo. You might elegantly establish this dish further and making yourself some keto avocado toast.

For this 10-minute keto toast dish, we've omitted the gluten-rich wheat flour. You'll use almond flour instead. Baking powder works in for yeast, which is a bonus offer for those of you who don't have yeast to use.

Ingredients.

- 1/3 cup (35 g) almond flour.
- 1/2 teaspoon (1 g) baking powder.
- 1/8 teaspoon (1 g) salt.
- One egg, blended.

- Tablespoons (37 ml) ghee, melted.

Instructions.

- Preheat oven to 200 F (400 C).
- Put all the bread components in a container and mix well.
- Microwave the mixture in the container and bake for 90 seconds.
- Let the bread cool for a few minutes, then take it out of the cup and cut it into four slices.
- Place the pieces on a baking sheet and place the toast in the oven for 4 minutes.
- Enjoy with some additional ghee.
- Some nights simply call for a toast, or you need quick recipes for breakfast. This recipe will not dissatisfy since you can make some Keto-friendly toast in just 10 minutes! Leading with your typical faves and take pleasure in it.

Keto Loaf of Bread [Gluten-Free, Dairy-Free]

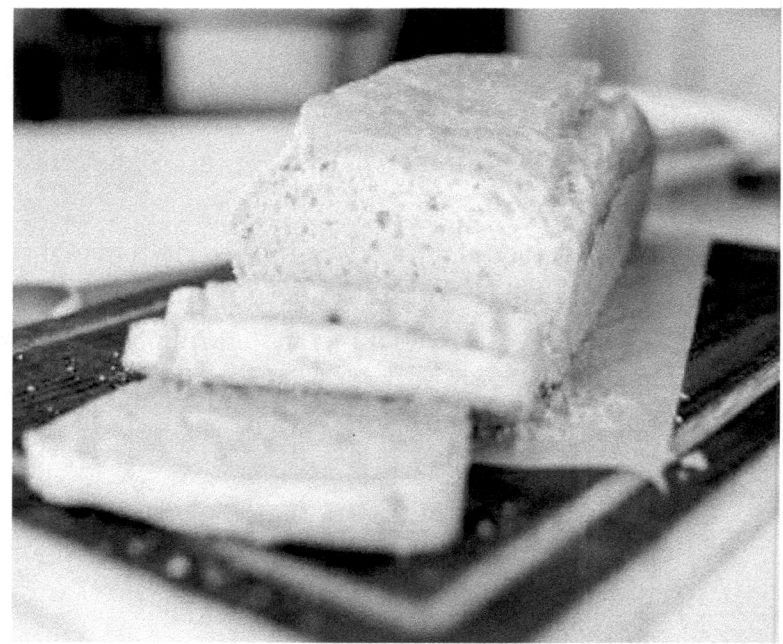

In fact, there are hundreds of methods for making fantastic bread. The problem is that most of them are very dependent on gluten. The key is to create a well-ventilated piece of bread. But there is another method.

Here, the recipe treatment technique is less like bread and more like cake. You have to knead and taste, this Keto bread starts with the dough. Baking soda and powder do all the work of filling bread with air, and voila.

How can I save my Keto bread?

Bread will be optimal to eat on the first day, and I would recommend doing it the day you want to use it. If you're going to do more, you may want to keep the bread in the refrigerator. So you will get 3-5 days of sweet bread as long as you allow the bread to warm to room temperature before consuming it. Anything above the five-day limit would be best to store all the extras in the freezer.

Ingredients

- 3 cups (360 g) almond flour
- 3 tablespoons whey protein powder (about 1 tablespoon).
- 1/2 cup + 2 tablespoons (150 ml) coconut oil.
- 1/4 cup (60 ml) coconut milk (canned).
- 3 beaten eggs.
- 2 teaspoons (9 g) baking powder.
- 1 teaspoon (5 g) baking soda.
- 1 tablespoon (3 g) Italian flavor.
- 1/4 teaspoon (1 g) salt.

Instructions.

- Preheat the oven to 150 F (150 C).
- Grease a bread pan (9 inches 5 inches) with olive oil or coconut oil.
- Combine all ingredients in a large bowl.
- Pour the dough into the pan and roll it out to fill as well.
- Bake for 60 minutes.
- Allow to cool, turn the pan over and cut into pieces with a bread knife.

Blueberry Loaf

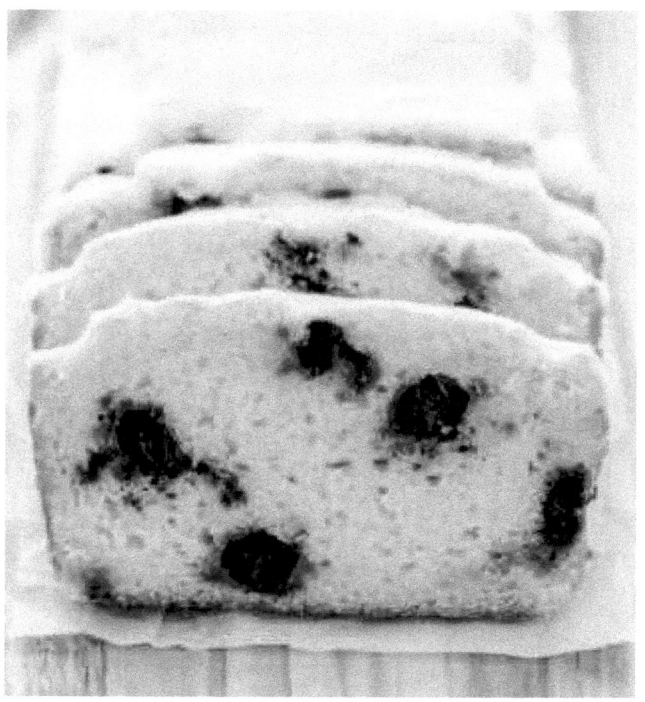

If you love blueberries, then you will wish to try this recipe. If you desire to make some delicious breakfast muffins, which will keep the whole family delighted, you can separate the mixture in the case of the bun.

Ingredients.

- 1 1/2 cups Almond Flour.
- 1 tablespoon Coconut Flour.
- 1 1/2 teaspoons baking powder.
- 7 tbsp Truvia (equivalent to one cup of sugar).
- 3 tablespoon oil.
- 4 tablespoon heavy cream.

- 1 teaspoon vanilla.
- 2 eggs.
- 100 grams of wild blueberries.

Instructions.

- Preheat oven to 300 degrees.
- Combine almond flour, coconut flour, baking powder, and six tablespoon Truvia with a whisk.
- Mix oil, whipping cream, and vanilla.
- Mix wet and dry ingredients together with a whisk. The batter will be thick!
- Wash off blueberries and include 1 tbsp of Truvia and stir.
- Put blueberries on carefully fold and top into the batter.
- Arrange a loaf pan with parchment paper and spread the batter in uniformly.
- Bake for 1 hour and 10 minutes ensuring to turn the loaf pan at about 30 mins in.
- Let cool totally in the pan.

Simple Loaf of Bread

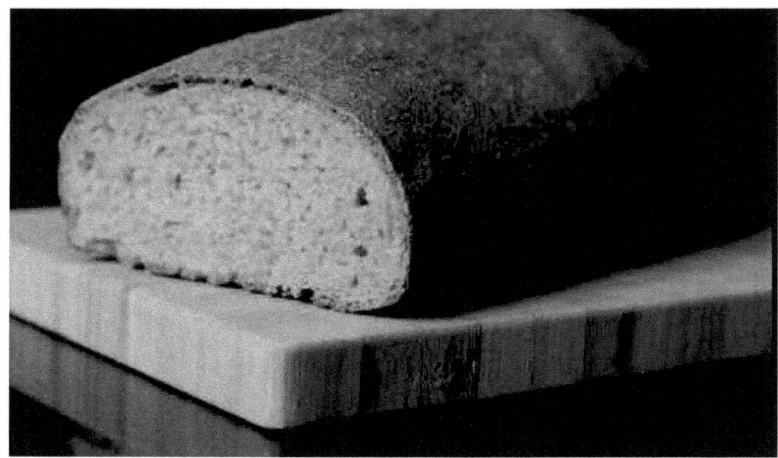

This dish gives a bread that can be used in any event where bread is typically served, with soups or as sandwiches for celebration nights, or you might include different components to alter it up.

For a Lighter Paleo Bread

If you desire the bread to be even lighter (or fluffier as I typically consider it), then you can include 1/3 cup pure whey protein powder and also 1/4 cup more almond milk.

Olive Oil or Coconut Oil?

When it comes to whether you ought to use olive oil or coconut oil in this dish, I try out both, and I like both (the olive oil version goes better with salted foods, and the coconut oil variation goes a bit better with sweeter foods).

Ingredients

- 3 cups (330 g) almond flour
- 1/2 cup + 2 tablespoons (150 ml) olive or coconut oil
- A quarter cup (60 mL) of almond milk (or water).
- 3 eggs
- 2 teaspoons (9 g) baking powder.
- 1 teaspoon (5 g) baking soda.
- 1/4 teaspoon (2 g) salt.

Instructions.

- Preheat the oven to 300F (149 C).
- Grease the bread (22.5 cm to 12.5 cm) (9 5 inches) (olive or coconut oil).
- Mix all the ingredients together.
- Place the dough in an ovenproof dish and spread it out to fill it evenly.
- Bake for 60 minutes.
- Leave to cool, turn the pan over and cut into pieces with a bread knife.

Keto Avocado Chocolate Bread.

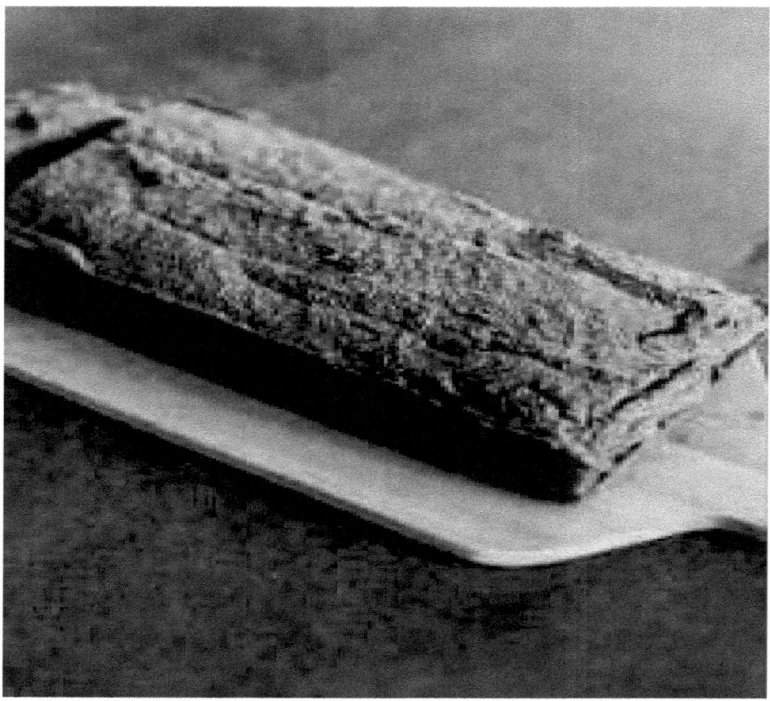

This bread is very scrumptious, healthy, with keto-friendly fats like avocado and coconut oil. It tastes nearly like a dessert because of the chocolate flavoring and the dash of stevia sweetener, but it's got the bread texture that you miss. So enjoy this for breakfast, lunch, as a treat, or as dessert!

Ingredients.

- 2 ripe avocados, mashed.
- 3 Tablespoons (45 ml) coconut oil.

- 3 eggs, blended.
- 2 cups (240 g) almond flour.
- 1/2 cup (48 g) cacao powder.
- 1 teaspoon (4 g) baking soda.
- 1/2 teaspoon (1 g) baking powder.
- 1 teaspoon (5 ml) vanilla extract.
- Stevia, to taste.
- Dash of salt.

Instructions.

- Preheat oven to 350 F (175 C).
- Mix whatever together.
- Place into a loaf pan.
- Bake for 40-45 minutes.

Sunflower Bread

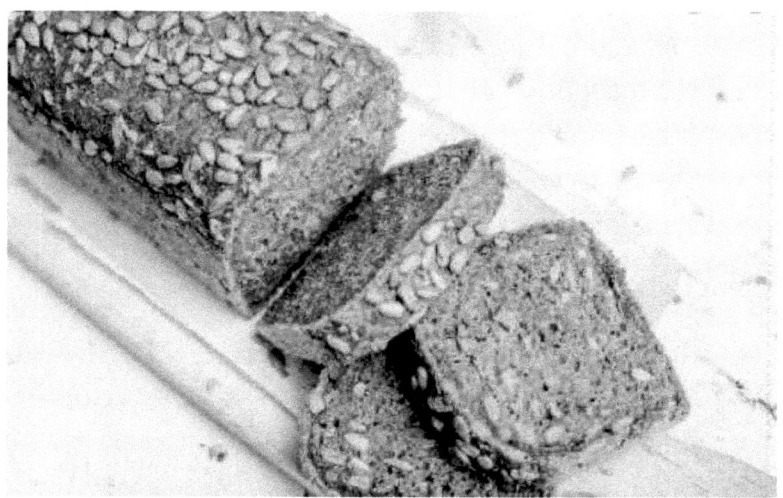

A fantastic alternative to regular dinner rolls. Makes regarding 15-- 20 rolls.

Ingredients

- 1 3/4 tsp (5 g) fresh yeast
- 1 1/4 cup (300 ml) water, space temperature level
- 3 cups (300 g) finely ground rye flour
- 2 1/2 cups (300 g) wheat flour
- 7 oz (200 g) rye sourdough starter
- 1 tbsp (15 g) salt
- 3 tablespoon (50 g) honey
- 2/3 cup (150 ml) sunflower seeds
- 1 tablespoon (10 g) cumin

Instructions

- Melt the yeast in a little of the water. Add all ingredients as well as mix well.
- Let the dough rise in a cozy place till it has actually increased in dimension. This will take 1 to 2 hrs.
- Shape the dough right into fifteen to twenty small rolls. Put them on a greased cooking sheet and also let them
- surge in a cozy area until doubled in dimension.
- Bake at 350 ° F (180 ° C) for about 10 minutes.
- Knead the dough after it has increased, and shape into a long roll.
- Cut the dough into fifteen to twenty items.
- They are forming right into rounded loaves as well as a place on a baking sheet to climb till doubled in dimension.

Keto Cornbread

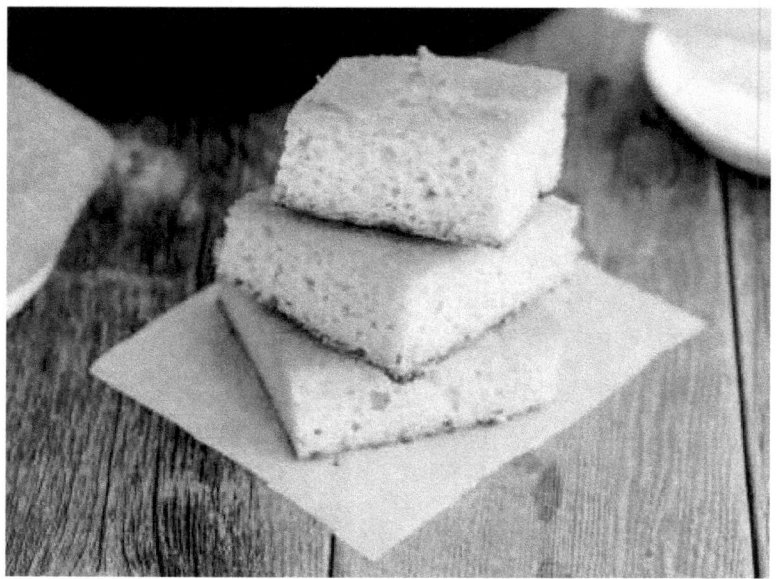

Paleo Cornbread that is low carb as well as keto! Made with coconut flour, it's nut-free as well as make the best bread for packing or clothing.

Ingredients

- 4 eggs
- 1 cup of water
- 2 Tablespoons apple cider vinegar
- 1/2 cup coconut flour
- 1/2 tsp garlic powder
- 1/4 cup coconut oil, melted
- 1/4 teaspoon sea salt, training course
- 1/2 teaspoon baking soda

Instructions

- Get your 4 eggs as well as bring to room temperature level. I crack mine in the blender as well as allow them rest for 20 mins or two.
- Add the apple cider vinegar, water, and 1/4 cup of melted coconut oil(not hot, so you don't cook the eggs), blend on for 30 seconds.
- After that, add in the coconut flour, garlic powder, salt, and cooking soda and also mix for one minute.
- Oil your baking tin with the 1 tsp coconut oil. I used two small mini loaves for this recipe.
- Pour the batter in your frying pans and also cook at 350 degrees for 40 - 45 mins.
- Non-compulsory, but if you want to get that great golden look, 1 minute before you take the bread out of the stove, scrub a tiny tsp of coconut oil on the top as well as broil on reduced until you obtain the color you want.
- Delight in! Yield:

10 Serving Size: 1

Quantity Per Serving: Calories: 109 Total Fat: 8g Saturated Fat: 6g Trans Fat: 0g Unsaturated Fat: 2G Cholesterol: 74mg Sodium: 149mg Carbohydrates: 4g Fiber: 1g Sugar: 1g Protein: 4g

Garlic Cauliflower Naan Bread Recipe

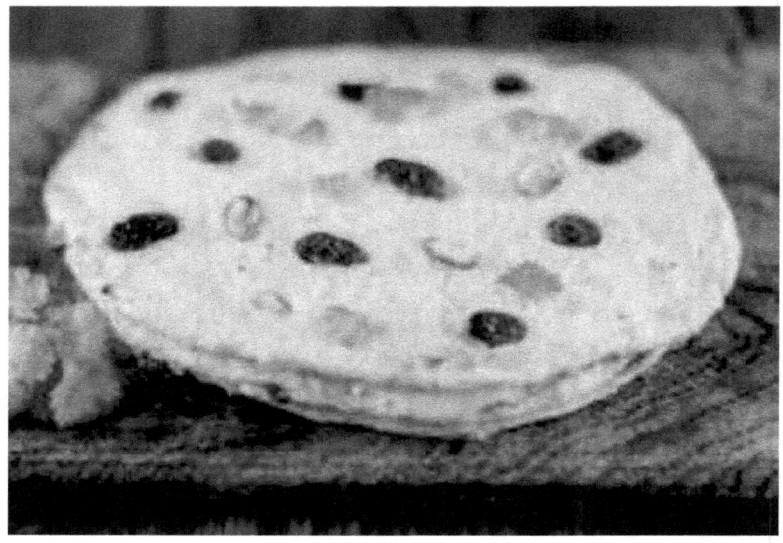

One of those dishes that I learned at the start was how to make focaccia bread that everyone will surely love. Plain bread can be beautiful, and the focaccia is so full of flavor and structure that you will always like it. Fortunately, this Keto focaccia bread plate is an excellent choice for a timeless plate filled with white flour and sugar. Using unusual ingredients, this recipe can make soft whole-grain bread. When baking bread, it should be smooth and slightly elastic.

Ingredients

- 1 cup (140 g) cauliflower
- 1/2 cup (64 g) arrow flour
- 1 tablespoon (7 g) garlic powder

- 2 tablespoons (30 ml) avocado oil (or olive oil).
- Salt to taste.

Instructions

- Preheat the oven to 450 F (230 C).
- Place the cauliflower flowers in a bowl with a little water and microwave on high power until smooth (check so they won't dissolve every 2 minutes). Sauté the herbs until they soften.
- Process the food (or use a blender) to turn the cauliflower flowers directly into the mash.
- Mix the cauliflower porridge with the butter-flour, garlic powder, avocado oil, and also the salt. Some prefer mixing and includes more garlic powder and salt to taste. Add the spring mixture.
- Press the dough directly on the flatbread with your hands, place it on baking paper, and bake for 15 minutes.
- Leave shiny and serve.

Trick

- Step 1:

Preheat your oven to 450 F (230 C) then make a dough by first cooking the cauliflower flowers to soften them. The simplest method is to place the cauliflower flowers directly in a container with a little water, as well as cook them in the microwave until they soften. You can also mate flowering plants until they soften. Then place the flowers directly in a blender or food processor and stir until they are combined.

65

- Step 2:

In a bowl, mix the cauliflower purée with the butter-flour, garlic powder, avocado oil (or olive oil), and also the salt.

- Step 3:

Knead directly into the elastic dough with your hands.

- Step 4:

Roll out the dough and place it on parchment paper. The dough should be about 1/3 inch (or 1 cm) thick.

- Step 5:

Bake 15 min.

- Step 6:

The bread should be smooth and lightly wiped along the edges. While tolerating the bread, it should be soft and slightly elastic. Let it cool down a bit and enjoy it.

Keto Flatbread Recipe With Nutritional Yeast

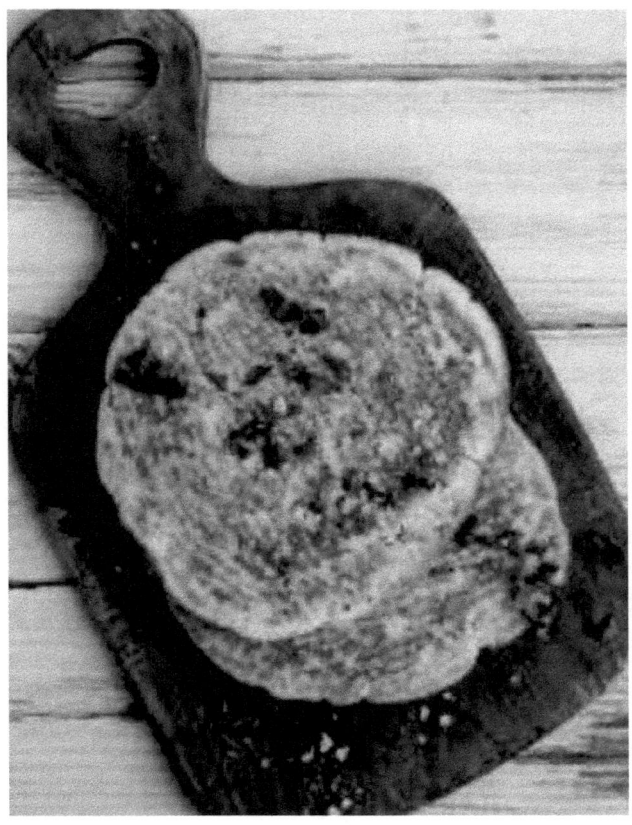

The ketogenic diet regimen is not the place for flour-filled, gluten-packed, or a carbohydrate loaded bread. There is an additional, better method.

Enjoying bread on the keto diet regimen requires alternative flours and a little creativity with the component list. All-purpose flour is out, but coconut flour, as well as almond flour, remain intact.

Below are just a couple of ideas of how to enjoy your flatbread:

- Egg and also bacon breakfast sandwich
- Set with soup or salad
- Leading with chicken or tuna salad
- Make a smoked cheese (be sure to examine the lactose content of your cheese of choice).
- Make a low-carb keto pizza (again, enjoy your macros).
- Consume with chicken and also avocado.
- Top with delicious grilled vegetables.
- Use them as fluffy taco coverings.

Ingredients.

- Half cup of (120 ml) unsweetened almond milk.
- 1 tablespoon (8 g) of dried out instant yeast or nutritional yeast flakes.
- 1.25 cup (140 g) coconut flour.
- 1 cup (120 g) almond flour.
- 2 teaspoons (4 g) baking powder.
- 1 tablespoon (10 g) garlic powder.
- 1 tsp (1 g) Italian spices.
- Dash of salt as well as pepper.
- 1 entire egg + 2 egg whites.

Instructions.

- Warm up the oven to 320 F (160 C).

- Warm the almond milk up in the microwave for 45 secs (or on the stove), after that whisk in the active dried yeast. Reserve to cool down somewhat. (The yeast will not be turned on without the existence of sugar, so this step is simply to add a tip of taste. If you have dietary yeast flakes, this will undoubtedly function similarly well, otherwise better).
- In a separate huge dish, combine the coconut flour, almond flour, cooking powder, garlic powder, Italian flavoring, salt, and pepper.
- Inspect the temperature of the warmed-up almond milk as you do not desire to add the eggs if it is still as well cozy (else the eggs will clamber). Blend in the egg as well as the two extra egg whites if you are satisfied it is not as well warm.
- Include the damp combination into the flour mix and also integrate well-making use of a wooden spoon. It should incorporate as a dough.
- Divide the dough into six tiny sections as well as shape right into a sphere and afterward flatten them. Roll or press right into a flat oval form (approx. 1/2-inch or 1 centimeter thick).
- Cook for 12-15 minutes.

Crunchy Rye Bread

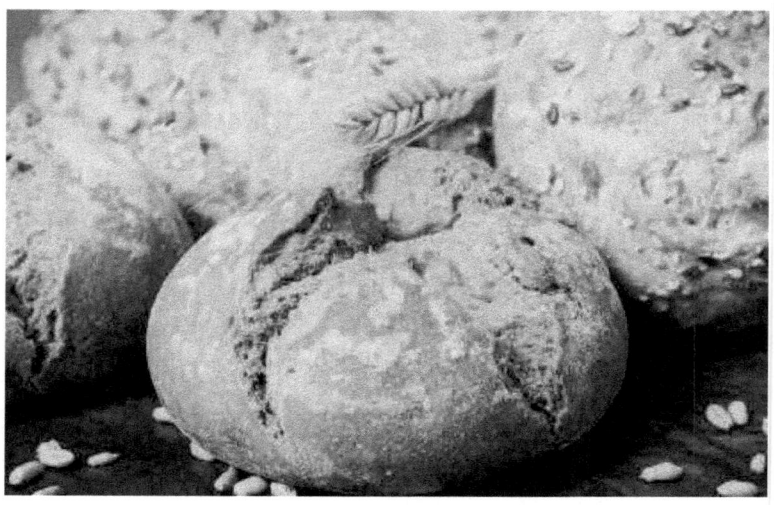

Makes regarding 20 biscuits

Ingredients

- 17 1/2 oz (500 g) rye sourdough starter made from entire wheat-rye flour
- 17 1/2 oz (500 g) wheat sourdough starter
- Five cups (500 g) fine rye flour
- 1/2 tablespoon (10 g) salt

Instructions

- Mix the ingredients well to allow the dough to rise for 2 hours.
- Roll the dough out as thinly as feasible. Cut into crackers and also place on a greased cooking sheet.

- Puncture with a fork to keep the bread from bubbling.
- Let the biscuits increase for 2-- 3 hours.
- Bake at 400 ° F(210 ° C) for approximately 10 minutes.

Beer Bread

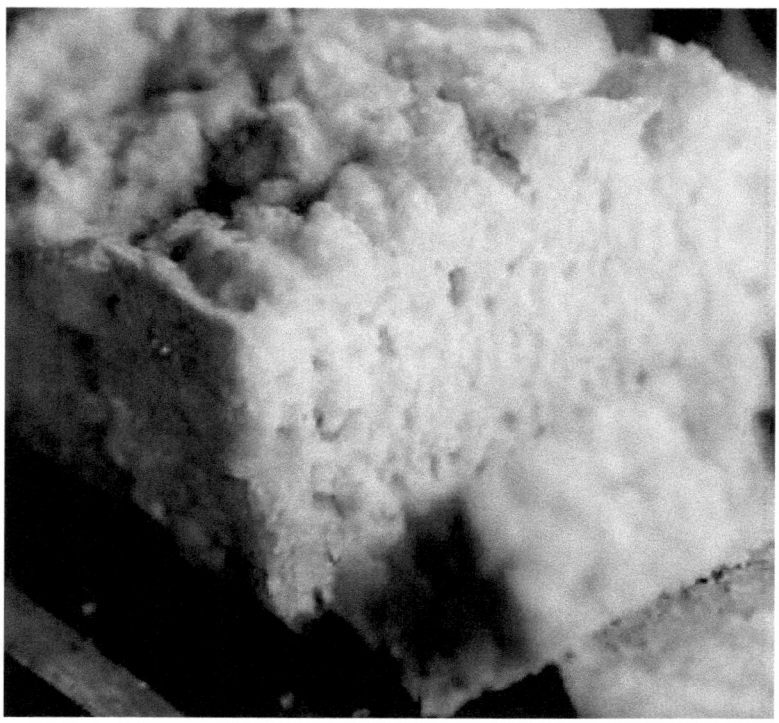

This is an acidic German bread. A product of cheese that produces a luxurious complement. Makes two loaves

Ingredients

- 1 1/4 cup (300 ml) beer, area temperature level
- 7 tsp (20 g) fresh yeast
- 1 tablespoon (15 g) salt
- 16 oz (450 g) rye sourdough starter
- 5 1/2 cups (700 g) entire wheat flour

Instructions

- Mix all the components, except for the flour. Add the flour a little by little and also blend well.
- Don't add all the flour simultaneously; check the dough to make sure that it is elastic before including even more flour. Knead well.
- Let the dough rest for about 15 mins. Knead well.
- Forming the dough right into two loaves and also let climb on a greased cooking sheet until it has roughly doubled in size. Spray a little flour over the bread.
- Firstly the Oven Temperature should be 475 ° F(250 ° C). Place the loaves in the oven as well as sprinkle a cup of water under it.
- Reduce the temperature level to 400 ° F(200 ° C). Bake the bread for 45 mins.

Tasty Crispy Bread

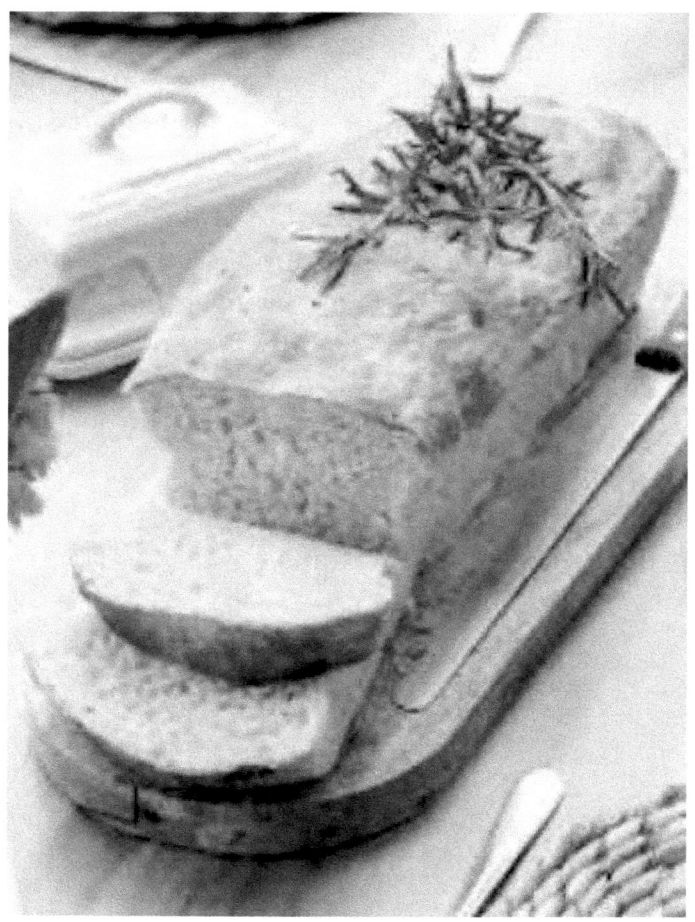

Makes 15 crackers Ingredients

- 1/2 oz (10 g) fresh yeast
- 1 2/3 cups (400 ml) cold water
- 3 1/2 oz (100 g) rye sourdough starter
- 3 1/2 oz (100 g) wheat sourdough starter

- 3 cups (300 g) whole rye flour
- 4 1/4 cups (550 g) wheat flour
- 1 tablespoon (15 g) salt
- 1/2 oz (15 g) anise
- Sea salt for covering

Instructions

- Liquify the yeast in the water as well as mix with the sourdough. Include the flour and knead thoroughly.
- Leave the dough for about 15 mins. Then add salt and also anise to the mixture.
- Place the dough in a bowl covered with plastic wrap. Let it rise in the fridge overnight.
- The following day, reduce the dough into fifteen portions. Roll each piece of dough out till it becomes thin as a biscuit.
- To keep the dough from sticking, gently flour the rolling pin. Sometimes turn the biscuit over to guarantee that you're spreading the mixture out effectively.
- Arrange the biscuits on a baking sheet covered in parchment paper. Puncture them with a fork
- Sprinkle with a little sea salt according to preference.
- Cook the biscuits at about 400 ° F (210 ° C) for 15 mins. Let the crackers dry on a cooling shelf

KETO
COOKIES

Keto Brioche

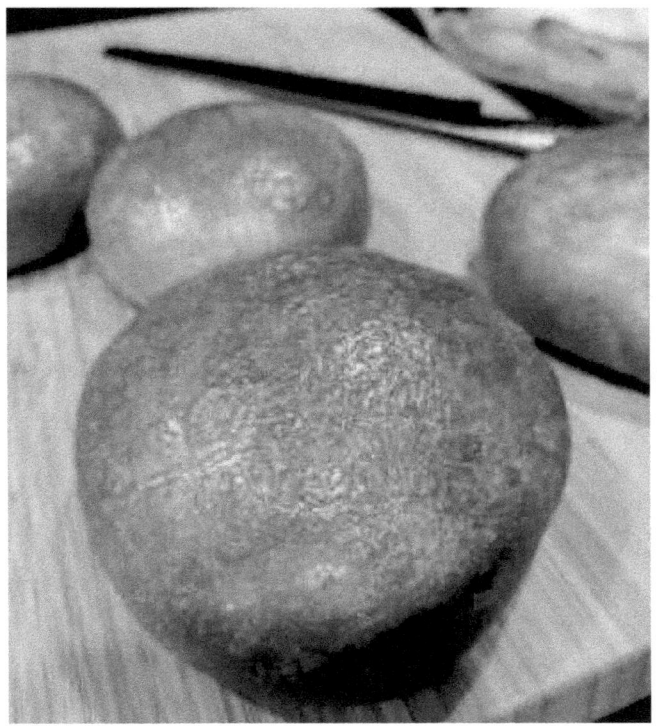

Makes about 20 rolls

Ingredients

- 3 1/2 oz (100 g) wheat sourdough starter
- 3 1/2 cups (450 g) wheat flour
- 2/3 cup (75 ml) milk, space temperature 5 1/4 tsp (15 g) fresh yeast
- Five eggs
- 2/3 cup (75 g) sugar
- 1 1/2 tbsp (25 g) salt
- 1 1/2 cup (350 g) unsalted butter, softened

- One egg for brushing

Instructions

- Mix the sourdough with fifty percent of the wheat flour, the milk, and the yeast. Allow the blend increase for 2HRs.
- Include all the components other than the butter and also mix extensively. Then, include the butter bit by bit in the 1/4 cup (50 g) each time and knead well.
- Use a clothe to cover it and let the dough increase for concerning 30 minutes.
- Form it into twenty little, smooth buns. Place them in cupcake mold and mildews and also let it rise until they increase in size.
- Brush the buns with the egg.
- Cook the brioche at 400 ° F (210 ° C) for about 10 minutes.

Cheesy Flax and Chia Seed Cracker Bread
(Low Carb and Gluten-Free)

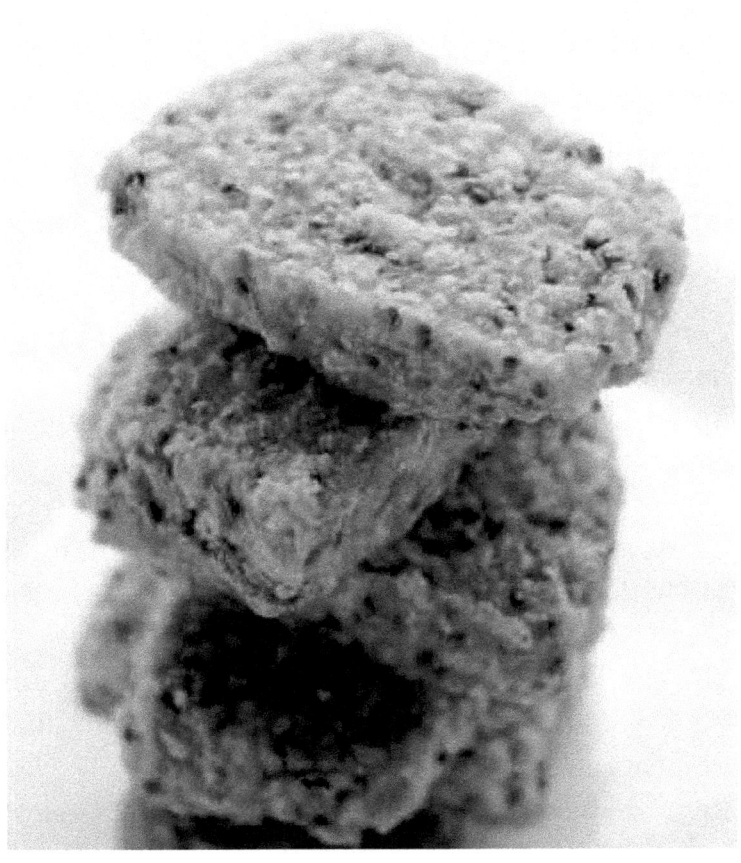

If you have been reducing your level of carbohydrate in your meal and you long for something crispy or chewy as an alternate for sandwich bread or also pizza dough, after that you just possibly be broken as well as hopeless enough to make and also eat these.

Ingredients.

- 1 1/2 oz ground flax.
- 2 Tbsp chia seeds (extremely suggest leaving out).
- 2 eggs.
- 1/2 oz shredded cheddar (use extra sharp).
- 1/2 tsp garlic powder.
- 1/2 tsp salt.
- 1/2 tsp pepper.

Instructions.

- Combine all active ingredients in a bowl and mix by hand up until a thick dough forms.
- Spray a sheet of foil or cling wrap with nonstick spray.
- Categorize the dough into a log shape with your hands as well as position on the cover. Roll it until it has to do with two lengthy and an inch of fifty percent in size.
- You can keep it around or press into a squared form. Pop right into the freezer for 5 mins till it firms up.
- Preheat the oven to 350 levels.
- Remove the dough from the fridge freezer and slice right into 1/4 to 1/2 inch thick pieces.
- Lay flat on a greased cookie sheet and also bake for 12-- 15 minutes till golden brownish.
- Remove it from the oven and allow to cool.

Wheat Buns

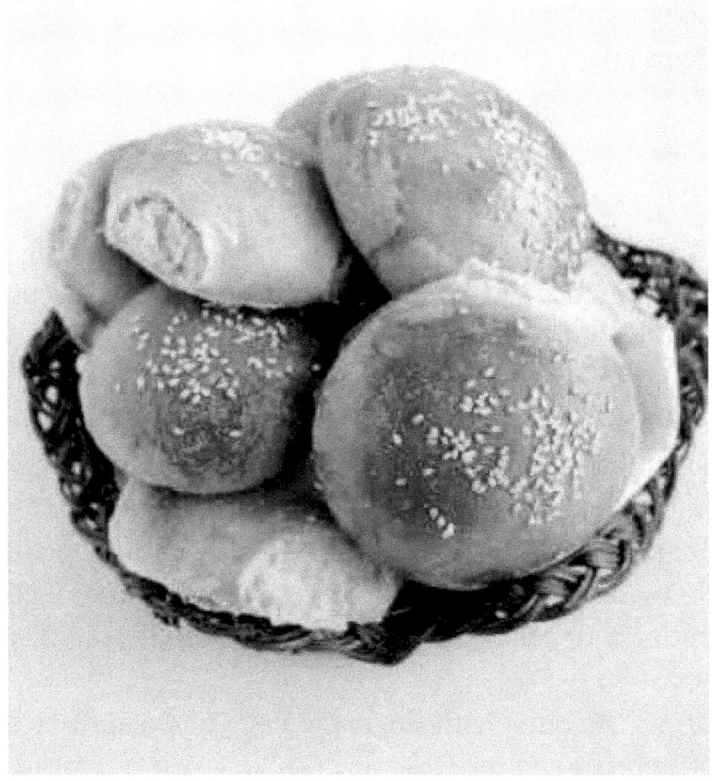

This dish can be used to make buns as well as knotted wreaths. Makes 35 buns

Ingredients

- 2 cups (500 ml) milk, room temperature level
- 1 3/4 oz (50 g) wheat sourdough starter
- 9 1/2 cups (1 1/4 kg) wheat flour
- 1 cup (200 g) butter
- 1/2 cup (75 g) fresh yeast
- 1/2 cup (165 g) white syrup

- 1/2 oz (15 g) ground cardamom
- 1 tsp (5 g) salt
- 1 egg for cleaning
- Pearl sugar for garnish

Instructions

- Mix 1 2/3 cup (400 ml) of the milk with the sourdough as well as half of the flour. Let surge for about 1 hour.
- Melt the butter and also allow cool.
- Dissolve the yeast in the staying milk. When done, add all the ingredients right into the initial dough as well as mix extensively. Knead until smooth.
- Shape the dough into thirty-five buns and position them on a greased cooking sheet. Let them climb under a towel up until they have actually doubled in size.
- Brush the buns with the beaten egg and a spray with a little pearl sugar—Bake at 400 ° F (210 ° C) for about 10 mins.

Keto Garlic Chia Crackers Recipe

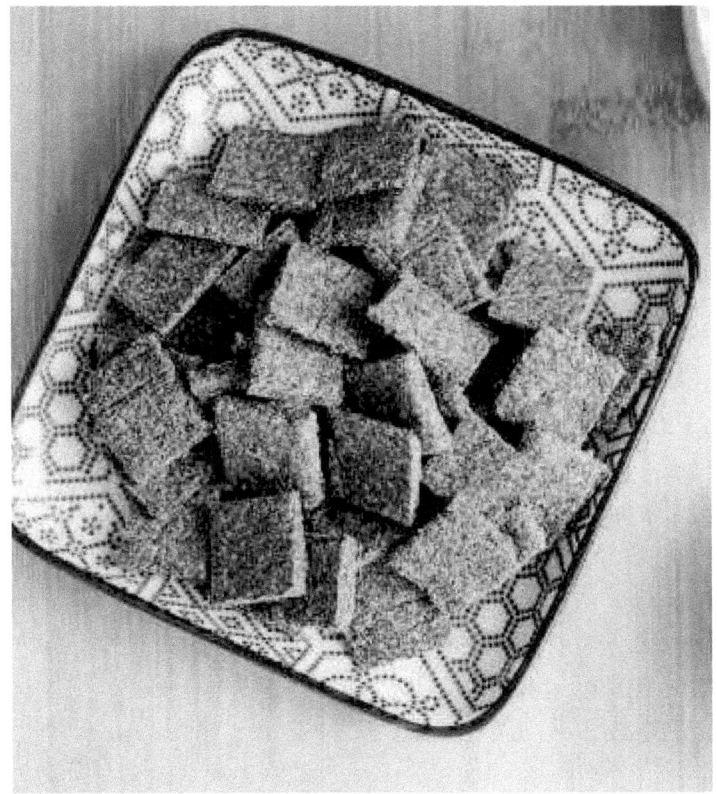

Crackers on a ketogenic diet? Not only is it feasible with this keto garlic chia crackers dish, but it's also easy. And they're downright delicious

You probably know most crackers can alter your keto diet. It's the cookies, the crackers, and even the pet crackers, which are relatively more cookie-like than anything. However, you can make them on your own.

This keto garlic chia crackers dish will not jeopardize your diet regimen, because they have exchanged a lot of the common active ingredients to suit your keto diet.

If you check the crackers ingredient label, you 'd possibly find sugar, high fructose corn syrup, white or all-purpose flour, soybean oil, and also some points you can't accommodate. The good news is, making delicious ketogenic snack worthy crackers requires none of those components. Instead, ground chia seeds develop the base, and garlic livens points up.

What to Pair With Keto Crackers

Take into consideration combining these biscuits with:

- Chili
- Soup
- Salads
- Almond butter
- Garlic dip

Ingredients

- Half cup (60 g) chia or flax meal (usage chia or flaxseed, and use a coffee grinder or a high blender to process into flour first).
- 1 egg, blended.
- 2 tablespoons chia seeds (24 g).
- 1 tbsp garlic powder (10 g).
- 1 teaspoon salt (5 g).

Instructions.

- Preheat the oven to 300F (150 C).
- Pour all the ingredients in a bowl to mix.
- Lay a piece of parchment paper on a flat surface. Put the dough on the paper and put another piece of parchment paper in addition to the mixture.
- Use a rolling pin to roll the dough to the desired density (about 0.2 cm thick).
- Carefully remove the piece of parchment paper and also use a sharp knife to mark the dough into small cookie squares.
- Place the parchment paper with the marked dough on a baking sheet and bake for 30 minutes.
- Break the cookies after 15 minutes and also return the cookies.
- Enjoy with the garlic sauce.

NOTES

All nutritional data is estimated and based on quantities per serving.

Nutrition :

Calories 123

Sugar 1g Fat

9g

Carbohydrates 8g

Fiber 5g

Protein 6g

Tasty Italian Crackers

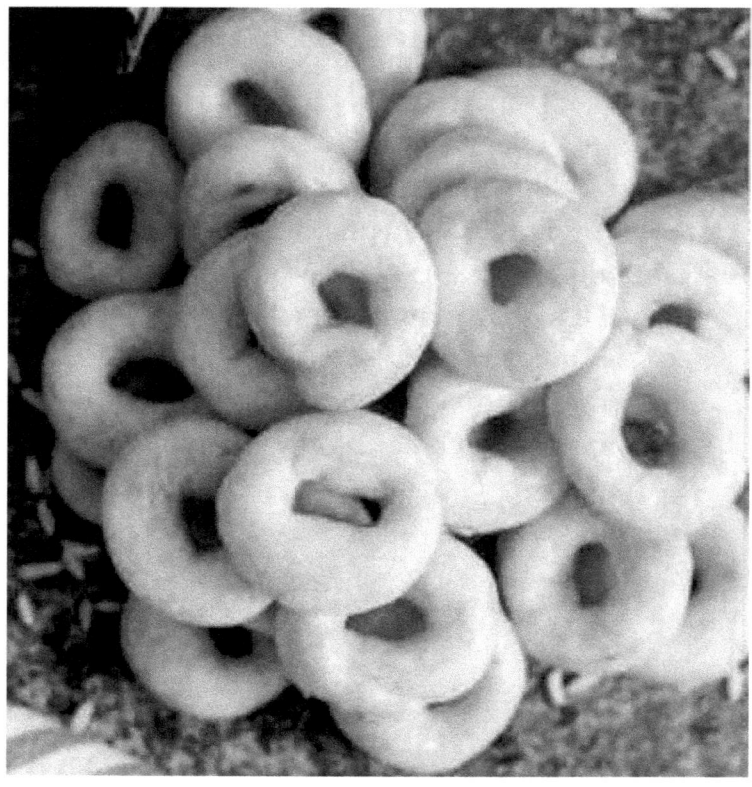

These biscuits are a simple means to obtain that experience back in a Paleo way. You can really make them in a range of flavors. Often you just require a little crunch in your life, and also these biscuits fill that void. With merely a handful of ingredients and within a half-hour, you can have self- made grain-free cookies. Use them to scoop up your favored dip or salsa, or eat them plain.

Ingredients.

- 1-1/2 cups (143 g) Almond Flour.
- 1 Egg.
- 2 Tbsp (30 ml) Olive Oil.
- 3/4 tsp (5 g) Salt.
- 1/4 tsp (0.5 g) Basil.
- 1/2 tsp (1 g) Thyme.
- 1/4 tsp (0.5 g) Oregano.
- 1/2 tsp (1 g) Onion Powder.
- 1/4 tsp (0.5 g) Garlic Powder.

Instructions.

- Preheat stove to 350 ° F(177 ° C).
- Mix all the active ingredients well to develop the dough.
- Shape dough into a lengthy rectangular log (use some foil or cling film to load the mixture tight) and also then reduced into slim slices (about 0.2 inches (0.5 cm) thick).
- Carefully place each slice onto a parchment paper-lined baking tray. It makes approx. 20-30 crackers, depending on dimension.
- Bake for 10-12 minutes.

Notes.

Substitutions: Italian spices can be used as opposed to basil, thyme, oregano, onion powder, and garlic powder if you do not have those readily available. Other nut flours can be used as opposed to almond flour (just food process the nuts using a mixer or blender right into an excellent meal).

Low Carb Panini

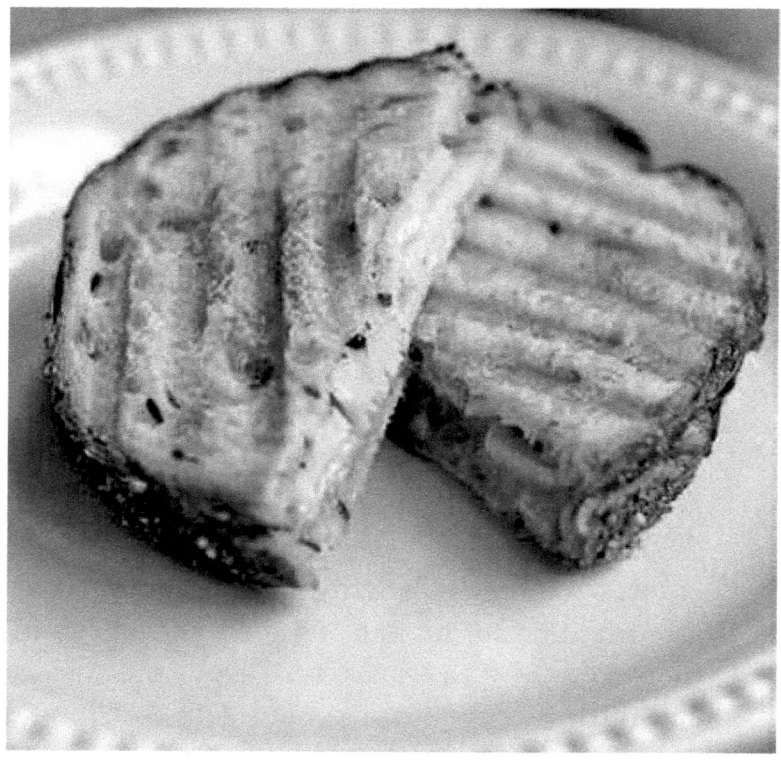

When one begins a low carbohydrate diet plan, one usually thinks that a panini sandwich will permanently be off-limits, together with bready foods. However, it's still pretty frustrating to face a world without panini.

You quickly find out that this is an incorrect impression that there are so many wonderful low carb foods available to you, consisting of bread, cookies, cakes, and muffins. It's impressive what you can do with a bag of almond flour, a stick of butter, and a desire to experiment.

Ingredients

- 1 recipe Low Carb Flatbread
- 2 tbsp Dijon mustard
- 2 tablespoon mayo
- 1/2 pound black forest ham
- 6 oz brie thinly sliced
- 1 medium green apple very thinly sliced
- Oil or melted butter for brushing beyond the sandwich

Instructions

- Preheat panini press.
- Cut bread into ten areas, then cut through the bready center of each section to get 2 flat, thin pieces.
- Add mustard and mayonnaise in a bowl for mixing.
- Pick up two matching sections of the bread and spread mustard/mayo combo on one side—layer with a few pieces of cheese, meat, and green apple.
- Brush each sandwich with oil or melted butter.
- Put on panini press and grill till bread is toasted and cheese is melted.

The look and texture of the flatbread are so good that no-one would presume they are actually healthy! Perfect for using to make sandwiches, these delicious treats can likewise be toasted, giving you an excellent version of panini. Position the dough between sheets of parchment, and this method will not stick to the rolling pin when you are rolling these out.

SECTION THREE
KETO PASTA RECIPES

Getting on the keto diet regimen indicates that appreciating a considerable dish of your average pasta is kind of out of the question. And, naturally, if you're on keto, you most likely think about diving into a dish of noodles all the damn time.

Thankfully, getting on keto does not have to indicate you can never ever, ever before, have pasta once again-- however you may need to get a little creative regarding it. Right here's what you need to learn about having pasta on keto, plus just how to rip off the system a little.

Easy Keto Lasagna

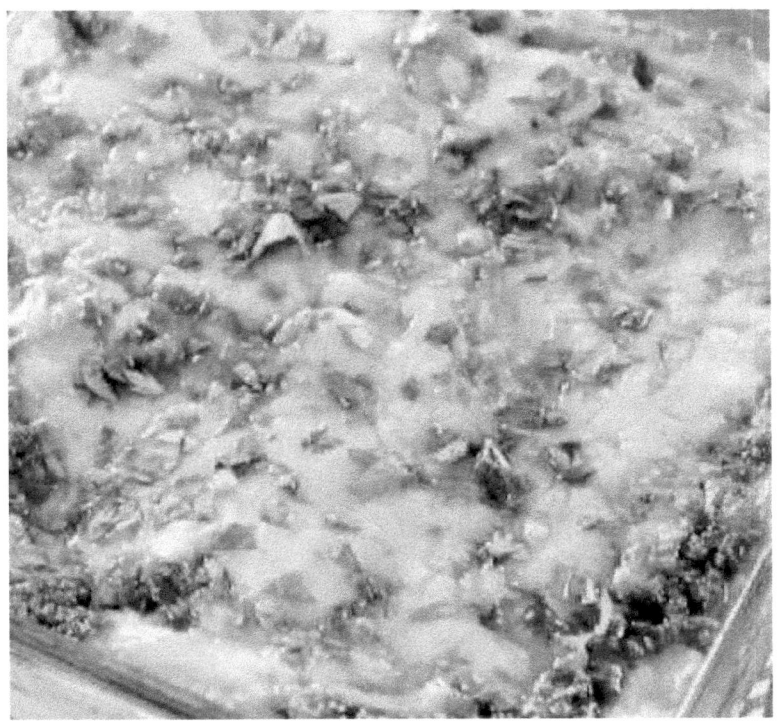

This easy keto lasagna will quickly turn into one of your new preferred dishes! It's tasty, abundant nutrients, and also easy layers! Lasagna usually takes a long period of time to make. However, I wished to still make a thick as well as a luscious dish that could be split and also continue to be tough. Cook Time: 25 minutes Total Time: 1 hr. 5 mins

Ingredients

- Meat sauce

- 1 pound ground beef
- 1 cup of raw spinach
- 1/2 cup low carbohydrate alfredo sauce
- ricotta blend
- 1/4 cup mozzarella cheese
- 1/4 cup grated parmesan
- 1/4 cup ricotta cheese
- 3 tbsp heavy cream
- 1/2 tsp Italian flavoring
- cauliflower layers
- 1 pound riced cauliflower, cooked
- 2 eggs
- 1/2 cup mozzarella
- 1/4 cup grated parmesan
- spices, to taste (I added garlic, salt, pepper, and Italian flavoring).

Steps.

- Preheat stove to 375.

For cauliflower

- Grate fresh cauliflower or use a ready bag of cauliflower rice. Drain all excess liquid using cheesecloth or towel.
- Mix eggs, mozzarella, grated Parmesan, and spices in a massive bowl with cauliflower rice.
- Spread cauliflower rice mixed as a pizza crust, about 1/4 -1/ 2 inch thick on a lined cooking sheet.
- Cook for 15 minutes or until golden brown, reserved.

For meat sauce (while cauliflower layer bakes).

- Brownish hamburger in a skillet, drain the fat and mix with alfredo sauce and raw spinach.
- Warm and proceed to cook until spinach is shriveled.

For ricotta filling.

- Mix ricotta, grated parmesan, heavy light whipping cream and flavoring together, set aside assembly.
- Oven at 375.
- Prepare an 8 × 8 baking meal with nonstick spray.
- Cut cauliflower sheet right into 2 halves as well as cut to fit the frying pan.
- Place one layer of cauliflower on the bottom of the pan (I needed to cut my own a little).
- Place fifty percent of meat sauce on top of layer, including a couple of extra spoons of alfredo if required.
- Include fifty percent of ricotta combination on top of the meat sauce layer as well as spray 1/4 cup mozzarella.
- Area 2Nd half of cauliflower layer as well as repeat last two previous steps with mozzarella on the top.
- Bake for 20 mins until gurgling after that broil for 3-5 minutes to brownish cheese.

Calories 514.1 Total carbohydrates (g) 4.9

Fiber (g) 0.3 Carbohydrates (g) 4.7 Protein (g) 21.1

Fat (g) 28.5 Total per serving (/ 6)

Keto Japanese Mushroom Pasta with Shirataki

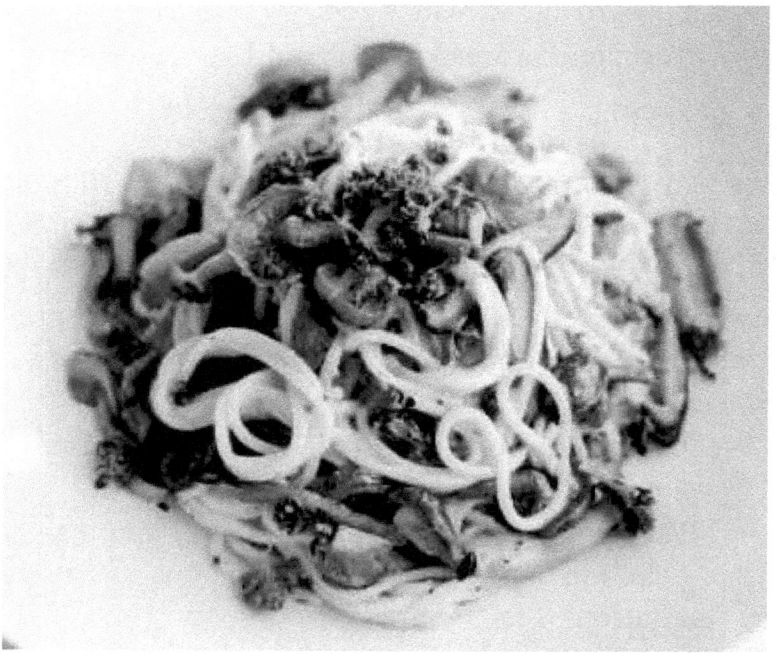

Ingredients

- 2 loads shirataki noodles
- 2 tbsp butter
- 2 cloves garlic
- 3 cups various mushrooms
- 1 teaspoon almond flour
- Pinch of dried parsley
- 3/4 thick tub cream
- Quarter tsp salt
- Quarter tsp pepper
- Olive oil
- Fresh parsley finely chopped, to garnish

Steps

- Prepare the shirataki by completely dry, frying them in a frying pan on tool warmth.
- Keep the warmth until they start making a whistling sound; this indicates the excess moisture leaving the noodles.
- Take it away from the pan and also set aside.
- Include your butter to the frypan and add the garlic. Cook for a min till great smelling.
- Pour the mushrooms in the frying pan after coating with oil and garlic. Cook for 5 minutes, mixing periodically, up until the mushrooms have ended up being a gorgeous golden shade.
- Take the mushrooms away from the pan, and leave the oil behind.
- Include the almond flour, dried out parsley and cream to the oil in the pan, and stir to combine.
- Include the salt and pepper to taste and also go on the warm for a couple of minutes.
- Ultimately, add the mushrooms and shirataki back right into the pan and combine.
- Serve piping warm with fresh parsley as well as enjoy it!

Notes

Nourishment Information (Approx): This dish makes two servings. Each serving has 4g web carbs (as pictured). Calories: 237kcal, Net carbs: 4g, Carbs: 14g, Fiber: 10g, Fat: 20g, Protein: 6g, Sugar: 3g

Cream Cheese Zucchini Spaghetti

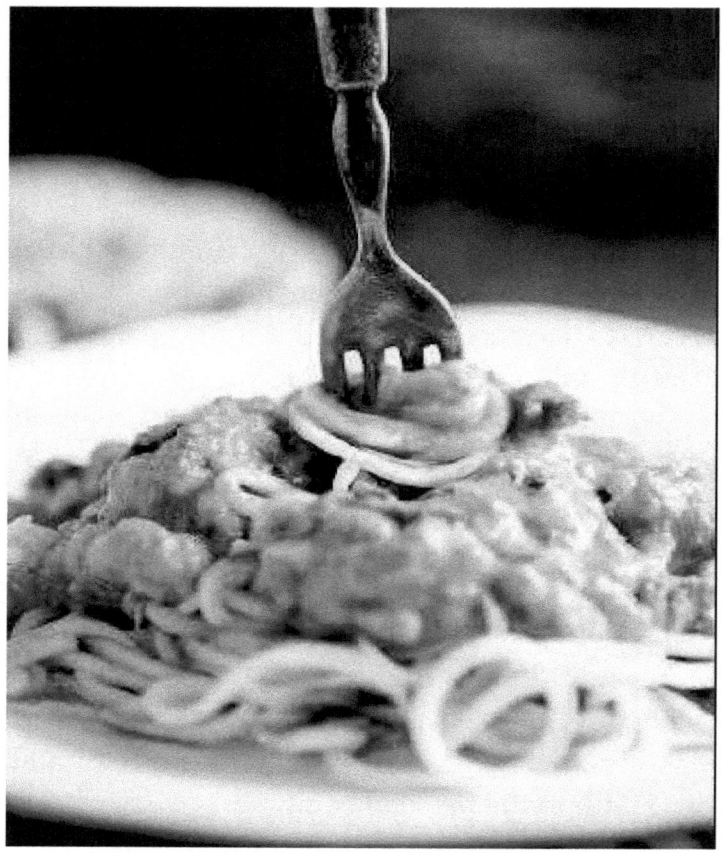

Are you considering a great low carb pasta, a lot of people have wanted an excellent spaghetti sauce, but tomatoes are simply naturally high in carbohydrates, and also when you start adding onions as well as garlic, you obtain a little even carb for my keto diet regimen. It's just three net carbohydrates per half-cup, and it's seriously some outstanding jarred sauce. Preparation Time is only 15 minutes with calories of 339 KCAL.

Ingredients

- 1 extra pound hamburger
- 15 ounces marinara sauce (see notes above).
- 4 ounces of cream cheese.
- 4 ounces sour cream.
- 8 zucchini.

Instructions.

- Brown the beef over medium heat, breaking it up as it cooks. When cooked, drain pipes the fat.
- Add the marinara sauce to the frying pan with the beef and warm over medium heat.
- Mix in the cream cheese as well as sour cream until melted and also velvety. Transform heat to low and also cover frying pan.
- Dry the zucchini and also cut the ends off. Utilizing a spiralizer, cut the zucchini into noodles.
- Place a considerable skillet over high heat. Spray with non-stick food preparation spray.
- Include the zoodles to the skillet (you might need to do this in batches) as well as cook, frequently throwing, till the zoodles reach the structure you prefer.

The longer you prepare them, the softer they get, but they additionally release a lot more water as they make it. Three minutes is just sufficient to take off a little bit of the crunch; however, keep them from releasing too much water. Offer sauce over the zoodles and enjoy it!

Calories: 339kcal (17%) Carbohydrates: 12 g (4%) Protein: 21 g (42%) Fat: 24 g (37%) Cholesterol: 77 mg (26%) Fiber: 3 g (13%) Sugar: 9 g (10%)

Pillowy-Soft Spinach & Ricotta Fried Ravioli

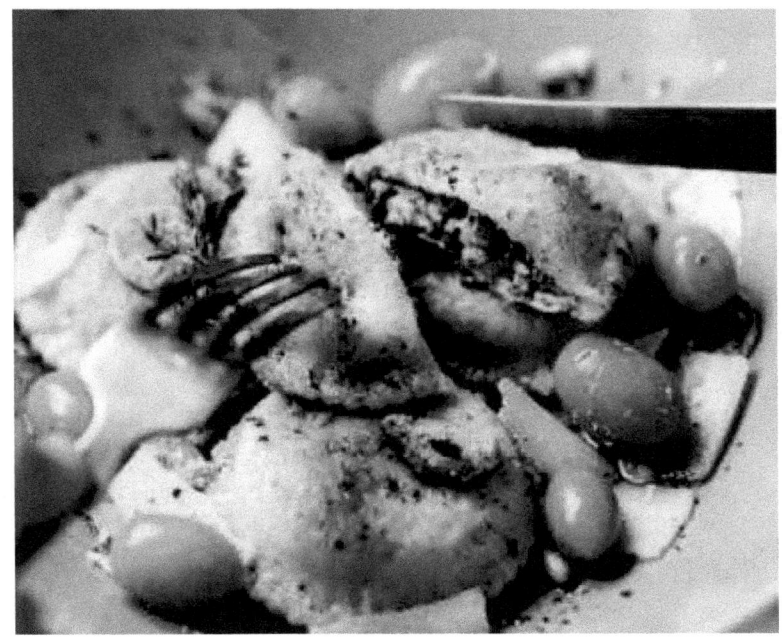

Spinach and ricotta keto pasta served with cherry tomatoes. These keto ravioli are a spinoff of grain-free keto tortillas. We need ingredients like almond flour, coconut flour, and a touch of xanthan gum, excluding the cooking powder.

Allergic to nuts? I've listened to excellent features of substituting the almond flour with sunflower seed dish or pumpkin seed meal from visitors. Color and also taste will be different, though.

Ingredients

The Keto Pasta Dough

- 96 g almond flour
- 24 g coconut flour
- 2 teaspoons xanthan gum tissue
- 1/4 teaspoon kosher salt depending upon whether pleasant or savory
- 2 tsp. apple cider vinegar
- 1 egg lightly beaten
- 3-5 teaspoons water

For The Ricotta & Spinach Filling:

- 1 tablespoon additional virgin olive oil for food preparation
- 250 g ricotta cheese
- 40 g Parmesan cheese newly grated
- 2 cloves garlic grated or ran through a press
- 400 g spinach
- 30 g pine nuts gently toasted
- 1/4 teaspoon fresh grated nutmeg
- kosher salt to preference
- black pepper freshly ground to preference
- 1 egg yolk
- 56 g grass-fed butter as needed
- 2 tablespoons added virgin olive oil
- 4 cloves garlic slivered
- 4 thyme springtimes
- cherry tomatoes to taste
- Parmesan cheese slivered

Instruction

For The Keto Pasta Dough

- Add almond flour, coconut flour, xanthan periodontal, and salt to a food processor. Beat until extensively combined.
- Pour in apple cider vinegar with the mixer running. Once it has actually dispersed equally, add the egg. Add water little by little, as needed, till the dough kinds right into a sphere. The mixture ought to be firm yet sticky to touch and also without any folds (which suggest the dough is dry, and also you need to add a little bit more water).
- Cover dough in stick film as well as massaged it through the plastic for a couple of mins. Consider it a little bit like a tension round. Leave the dough to rest for 15 minutes at space temperature and also place in the fridge for 45 minutes (as well as approximately five days).

For The Ricotta & Spinach Filling:

- Heat up olive oil in a frying pan or pan over tool heat. Include garlic and also sauté briefly up until gold. Include spinach and refuse the warmth. Once wilted, eject excess fluid, transfer it to the board, and chop it. Permit to cool.
- Combine spinach with ricotta, grated Parmesan cheese, toasted nuts, and newly grated nutmeg. Season to taste with salt and also freshly ground pepper to preference. Mix in egg yolk.

To Accumulate The Ravioli

- Use a pasta device or a tortilla press to roll out the pasta to its thinnest point (in between parchment paper). You can additionally use a moving pin, but it'll take a little bit much longer.
- Heap about a tablespoon of filling up onto the dough. Press the 2Nd item over it and push down around the sides to seal, removing any kind of air bubbles. The dough will certainly be sticky, so no egg wash is required. Trim the sides near the filling using a cookie cutter (or pizza cutter/knife/glass). Sort all the ravioli on a cooking tray and also freeze for 15 mins before cooking.

For The Thyme-Butter Sauce

- Heat up butter and oil in a frying pan or pan over low heat. When cozy, add in garlic slivers and thyme. When the garlic begins to brown, include cooled ravioli.
- Cook pasta in the butter until gold throughout, a min or two on each side. If the garlic bits begin to brownish way too much, you'll intend to pull them out (do not throw out).
- Serve immediately over a bed of cherry tomatoes and topped with slivered parmesan as well as the crunchy garlic bits (opt-out if garlic isn't your point).

Techniques

The real technique right here is to get the keto pasta dough good and also slim.

1. Present the dough between parchment paper

This is easiest done when making use of either a tortilla press (actors iron ones are the best) or real pasta equipment. Putting the spinach as well as ricotta dental filling over the keto pasta dough

2. Include filling

Load roughly a tbsp of filling onto the dough. Press the 2Nd item over it and also push around the sides to seal, eliminating any air bubbles. The mixture will undoubtedly be sticky, so no egg wash is required.

3. Trim

I just used a cookie cutter below, but feel free to utilize whatever drifts your watercraft. Simply keep in mind that you'll intend to trim the edges near to the dental filling.

4. Freeze

You'll intend to ice up the pasta for 15 minutes before cooking. And indeed, you can go on as well as freeze them too, however, thaw them out a little before food preparation. You'll likewise want to prepare these people always in a little olive oil or butter, never ever in water (they'll simply be mushy).

Think of these grain complimentary and keto pasta as pillowy-soft attacks from heaven. Filled with spinach, ricotta, and also toasted want nuts, they're Chicken fried in a clove of garlic and also thyme-infused brownish butter for an impressive outcome.

NOTES

Feel free to go on as well as ice up the ravioli, but you'll wish to thaw them out a little prior to food preparation. This dish yields 20 x 2 1/2 inch pasta. Nourishment facts below were estimated per ravioli with the dental filling, so a serving of 4 pieces is 6g net carbs.

Amount Per Serving   Calories 88

Fat 6g (9%)   Saturated Fat 2G (10%)   Cholesterol 25mg (8%)   Sodium 93mg (4%)   Potassium 138mg (4%)

Carbohydrates 3g (1%)   Fiber 1.5g (6%)   Protein 4g (8%)

Keto Ricotta Gnocchi

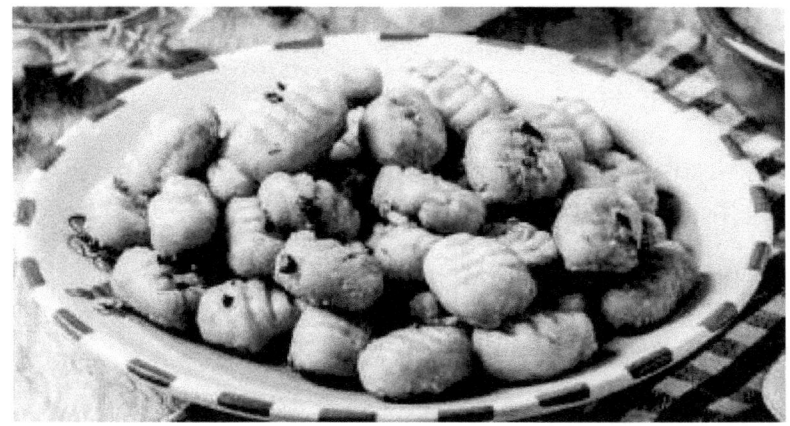

This keto ricotta gnocchi also requires a mixture of almond flour, coconut flour as well as a touch of xanthan gum tissue. All the ingredients are blended till they develop a (sticky!) sphere, refrigerated for an hour, formed right into rounds, flattened with a fork, as well as cooked in sage butter.

This gluten-free and keto ricotta gnocchi are pillowy-soft, unbelievably aromatic, and also paired with a refreshingly straightforward Mediterranean yogurt sauce.

Ingredients.

For The Keto Ricotta Gnocchi.

- 128 g almond flour.
- 14 g coconut flour.
- 2 teaspoons xanthan gum tissue.
- 210 g ricotta cheese.

- 75 g Parmesan cheese freshly grated.
- Kosher salt to preference.
- 1 egg lightly defeated.
-

For The Sage Butter.

- 3-4 tablespoons grass-fed butter as required.
- 1 Tsp of extra virgin olive oil.
- Two garlic *cut it thinly*
- 8-10 sage leaves.
- Black pepper freshly ground to taste.
-

For The Mediterranean Yogurt Sauce.

- 140 g Greek-style yogurt.
- 1 clove garlic went through a press.
- 2 tsp. Additional virgin olive oil.
- 1/2 -1 teaspoon red wine vinegar to preference.
- Kosher salt.
- Black pepper newly ground to preference.

Serving Suggestions.

- Spinach steamed.
- Cherry tomatoes.

Steps.

FOR THE KETO RICOTTA GNOCCHI.

- Add almond flour, coconut flour as well as xanthan periodontal to the bowl and also blend up until thoroughly integrated.
- Add ricotta and also parmesan to a big dish and combine with a spoon until well incorporated.
- Add the flour to the mixture and also blend well. Add salt for taste and mix in the egg. The dough must be sticky but form right into a ball conveniently. If it does not (different wetness degrees in cheese, etc.), feel free to add in more almond flour a little at once.
- Wrap in stick film (saran wrap) as well as refrigerate for at the very least an hr.
- Remove dough from the refrigerator and also type right into rounds (approximately 1 inch huge). The mixture will undoubtedly be soft and even still lightly sticky, yet need to develop right into rounds effortlessly.
- Put in a tray and also compress it down using a fork to lightly flatten them.
- Freeze for 15 minutes before frying, and the gnocchi can be iced up now for up to 2 months.
- Heat up butter as well as oil in a skillet or frying pan over medium/low heat.
- Once warm, add in garlic bits and sage leaves. When the garlic is simply lightly gold, include the chilled gnocchi flat-side down along some fresh ground black pepper.
- Move the frying pan around to keep them from sticking, basting them throughout the food preparation. They will be delicate, so handle with

care. When all set, the bottom will have developed a deeply golden crust, about 4-5 minutes.

- Serve as soon as possible and top with a bed of steamed spinach, yogurt sauce, and a handful of cherry tomatoes (optional).

For The Mediterranean Yogurt Sauce.

- Mix all components together as well as cold up until required.

NOTES.

Feel free to go on as well as ice up the gnocchi, however, you'll intend to thaw them out somewhat before cooking. Keep in mind that nourishment facts were estimated per 80g offering of the gnocchi only, and the recipe returns 6 portions.

Calories: 315kcal | Carbohydrates: 8g Protein: 13g Fat: 26g Saturated fats: 9g | Trans fat: 0g | Cholesterol: 65mg Sodium: 403 mg Potassium: 55 mg Fiber: 4g Sugar: 1g | Vitamin A: 450 IU Vitamin C: 0.7 mg Calcium: 236 mg Iron: 1.3mg Net carbohydrates: 4 g

KETOGENIC PASTA RECIPES WITH MEAT

Keto Crockpot Beef Stroganoff

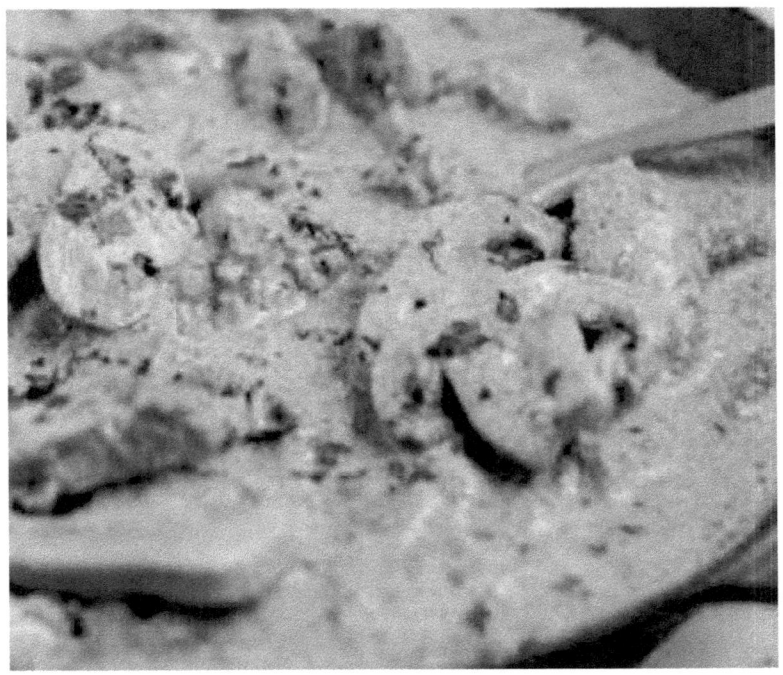

This lip-smacking beef stroganoff recipe will positively be contributing to your keto cookbook, with hearty components as well as a warming satisfaction after eating. Typical stroganoff has a whole lot of non-keto active ingredients which can be conveniently switched out and still yield ultra-yummy results. Popping active ingredients into a crockpot is so straightforward, you'll certainly intend to attempt this dish at the very least once!

After preparing your beef as well as vegetables in the slow stove with this tasty bone brew, you'll get an abundant and flavorful dish. Top it with coconut milk and Dijon mustard sauce and leading place on top of Keto pasta to serve.

Preparation Time: 10 mins; Cook Time: 8 hours; Yield: 6 servings; Category: Dinner; Cuisine: Russian.

Ingredients

- 2 lbs. Beef roast, cut into tiny strips (or utilize Chicken busts).
- 1 big onion, chopped.
- 4 cloves garlic, diced.
- 3 Tablespoons parsley, cut.
- 1 cup (100 g) white mushrooms, cut (approx. 10 mushrooms).
- 2 cups (480 ml) canned mushroom chicken bone broth.
- Salt and pepper.

To serve:

- 1 cucumber, peeled into lengthy large strips.
- Half cup (120 ml) of coconut milk/cream.
- 3 tablespoons (45 ml) Dijon mustard.
- Salt.
- Parsley for garnish.

DIRECTIONS.

- Add the beef, onion, garlic, mushrooms, beef broth, black pepper, as well as salt right into a slow stove/ crockpot as well as cook on a reduced temperature level for approx. 6-8 hours. The beef ought to be really tender when it's done.
- After the beef is done, mix right into the sluggish cooker pot the coconut cream, Dijon mustard, salt to preference.
- Place the cucumber noodles right into a dish. Top with the beef stroganoff. Garnish with the remaining parsley.

NOTES.

All nutritional data are estimated as well as based upon per offering quantities. Net Carbs: 3 g.

NUTRITION.

They were serving Size: 1 bowl Calories: 462 Sugar: 2 g Saturated Fat: 36 g Carbohydrates: 4 g Fiber: 1 g Protein: 26 g.

Spaghetti Squash Bolognese

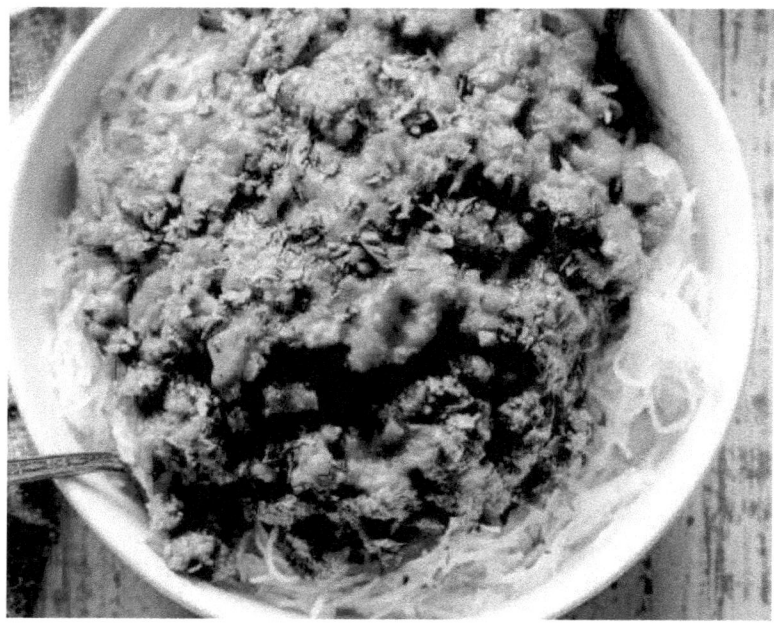

Using pasta squash is a healthy and balanced alternative to traditional pasta and can be eaten using the same method. This reduced carbohydrate dish is an excellent method to present squash into your kids' diet plan, and they might also find out to like it as much as they love pasta. If you include the basil at the end of the cooking time, it aids in preserving the complete quality of the taste.

This tasty Paleo and Keto spaghetti squash Bolognese recipe are easy to cook and also makes a terrific dinner for the entire family. It's gluten-free and makes use of spaghetti squash as opposed to regular wheat kinds of pasta.

You can transform the meat in this dish to ground turkey or chicken if you choose (although those meats are generally lower in fat, so may not be desirable if you're on a high-fat ketogenic diet).

When you make this pastas squash dish, make sure to include the fresh diced garlic as well as diced basil leaves as they really give the meal a lot of flavors. Adding in those components towards completion of the dish makes those flavors stay in the meal better.

Ingredients

- 1 large pasta squash (approx. 5 pounds).
- 2 lb. (908 g) ground or minced beef.
- 1 onion, diced.
- 1 14.5 oz (410 g) can of diced tomato.
- 1 cup (40 g) fresh basil, carefully sliced.
- 8 cloves of garlic, peeled off and minced.
- 1/4 cup (60 ml) coconut oil to cook the beef with.
- 2 Tablespoons (30 ml) coconut oil to prepare the spaghetti squash.
- Salt and pepper to taste.

Instructions.

- Place 1/4 cup of coconut oil into a big pot and also sauté the diced onion in the oil above heat.
- Add the hamburger to the pot once the onions transform transparent.
- When the meat is browned, add the diced tomatoes and turn down the warm. Simmer with the lid on for 30 mins (simmer for 1 hr. if you have time).

113

- Stir regularly to make sure it's not sticking to an all-time low of the pot.
- On the other hand, slice a pasta squash in half, remove the seeds, add them within with a thin layer of coconut oil (you can use your hands to do this), cover with a paper towel to avoid splattering, and microwave each spaghetti squash fifty percent for 6- 7 minutes on high power.
- Alternatively, you can cook the coconut oil covered pasta squash fifty percent in the stove at 375 F (190 C) for 45 mins.
- Utilize a fork to scratch out the pasta squash strands and split them between 4 plates.
- Add the basil, garlic, salt, and also pepper to taste to the meat sauce, cook for five more minutes.

NOTES.

All dietary data are estimated and based on per serving amounts. Net Carbs: 9 g.

NUTRITION.

Calories: 440 Sugar: 5 g Fat: 34 g Carbohydrates: 12 g Fiber: 3 g Protein: 20 g.

Asian Garlic Beef Noodles

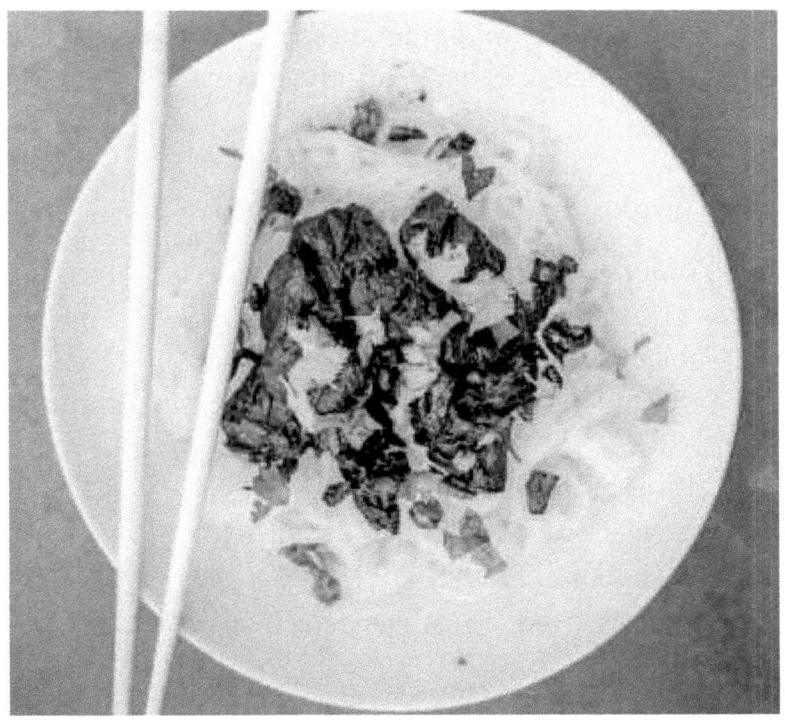

Ginger and also garlic are the most usual essential active ingredients in Asian cuisine, and also they make this dish taste so excellent! This keto noodle dish is quite fast to make, serving you a quick, tasty meal for unforeseen supper visitors or after a busy day at the workplace. The fragrances from the beef will undoubtedly make your mouth water! Try making use of red onion instead of a gentler, somewhat sweeter preference. One of the very best aspects of several oriental recipes is just how fast they are to make.

Take this garlic beef noodles recipe, for instance. It's likewise incredibly delicious with garlic, ginger, as well as cilantro for seasoning. For the noodles, you can make use of zucchini noodles, cucumber noodles, or shirataki noodles for a complete series of Paleo pasta alternatives.

Ingredients

- 1/2 onion, sliced
- 10 oz (300 g) beef, cubed or sliced
- 2 Tablespoons avocado oil (or coconut oil).
- 2 Tablespoons tamari sauce (usage coconut aminos for AIP).
- 10 cloves garlic, diced.
- 1 huge piece of fresh ginger, diced.
- 2 Tablespoons cilantro, cut (for garnish).
- 1 zucchini, shredded, or use a pack of shirataki noodles.

Steps

- Cut the onion upright into thin slices.
- Sauté the onions in some avocado oil (or coconut oil, although it favors the taste of avocado oil when blended with tamari sauce or coconut oil.
- Add the beef dices to the frying pan. You can make use of stew meat or any other beef chopped into tiny cubes. You can additionally use small pieces of meat if you have time to slice it.
- Add the tamari sauce or coconut oil to the frying pan.

- Place a lid on the frying pan. This will get the beef to prepare faster If you are making use of very finely sliced meat, it will undoubtedly cook quicker so you can skip this action.
- Fresh ginger, and garlic cloves, are the keystone of this dish. So be really liberal with them. Peel and also about slice up the ginger as well as garlic.
- Add the garlic and also ginger to the pan when the beef is cooked sufficiently.

NOTES.

All dietary information is estimated as well as based upon per serving quantities.

NUTRITION.

Calories: 620 Sugar: 0 g Fat: 50 g Carbohydrates: 5 g Fiber: 0 g Protein: 37 g.

Eggplant Lasagna

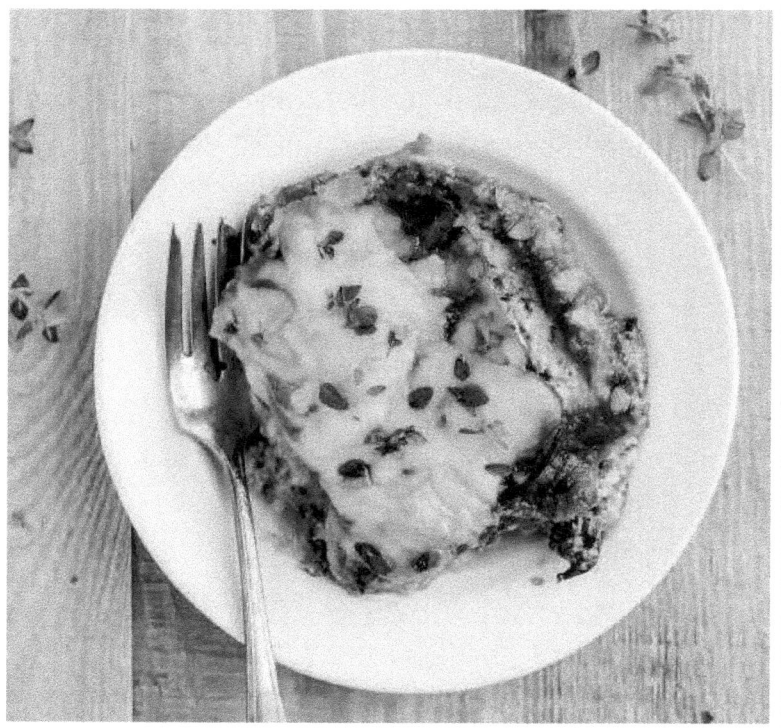

We've examined this lasagna recipe a ton of different ways, and we've paleo field it a bunch by extracting the sugar, the wheat-filled pasta sheet pasta, the Italian sausage (which sometimes contains additives or sugar), and the three sorts of cheese!

This Paleo lasagna recipe uses pieces of steamed eggplants as the lasagna pasta. I've seen various other options (e.g., spinach leaves, zucchini, broccoli), but I like eggplants as it does not include much of its taste and is the right sort of color for pasta. Nonetheless, if you prefer to utilize something else, after that, you can just replace the eggplants in this recipe with your option of "paleo pasta."

You can mix of beef and pork in this Paleo pasta dish. This mix worked most effectively; however, you can change the blend with the same quantity of meat of your deciding on.

This Paleo lasagna recipe was so good I pretty much forgot that there was no cheese in it! To make it look a bit prettier, I split a few prompts top of the pasta. You can instead just make use of egg whites to give it more of a cheese look or else usage something like soaked cashews blended.

Preparation Time: 15 mins; Cook Time: 1 hour 50 minutes Yield: 8 portions Category: Lunch, Dinner Cuisine: Italian.

Ingredients.

- 3/4 lb. Ground pork (or utilize meat of your choice).
- 3/4 pound hamburger (or use meat of your optional).
- 1 little onion, diced.
- 4 cloves garlic, smashed.
- 1 (28 oz) can be diced of smashed tomatoes.
- 2 (6 oz) canisters of tomato paste.
- 2 Tablespoons fresh basil, finely sliced.
- 6 Tablespoons fresh parsley, carefully sliced.
- 1 Tablespoon fresh oregano, carefully sliced.
- 1 Tablespoon fresh thyme, carefully chopped.
- 1 teaspoon fennel seeds.
- 2 eggs, blended.
- 2 Tablespoons coconut oil.
- Salt to preference.

- 1 huge eggplant (or 2 Japanese eggplants), cut into thin pieces.
- 3 eggs for topping (optional).
- 3 Tablespoons of salt for boiling eggplants.

Instructions.

- Add the 2 tbsps of coconut oil right into a big stockpot. Include the ground meat and also the minced onion. Cook up until the meat browns, and the onion turns clear.
- Then include the smashed tomatoes, tomato paste, natural herbs, fennel seeds, and smashed garlic.
- Prepare on a reduced simmer with the lid on for 45 mins.
- Mix regularly to ensure nothing adheres to the bottom of the pot.
- Preheat the stove to 375F and also boil a pot of water. Include the 3 tbsps. Of salt into the boiling water, after that, add in the eggplant pieces.
- Boil for 2-3 minutes, then remove and position it cold water (if your slices are thicker, after that you may need to boil for longer the eggplant ought to soften to ensure that you can suffice with a fork rather quickly).
- Add in the whisked eggs right into the meat mix and also stir slowly to mix the eggs in.
- Cook the meat combination for 10 mins more and afterward include salt to preference.
- Put half of the meat mixture right into an all-time low of a 13 by 9-inch lasagna pan or a similar baking

frying pan. Top with half the pieces of steamed eggplants.

- After that, put the other half of the egg mixture on top of the eggplant pieces, as well as top that meat layer with the rest of the eggplant slices.
- Cover the tray with aluminum foil as well as cook for 30 minutes.
- Get rid of the aluminum foil and fracture the 3 agitate top (optional).
- Bake for 15-20 more minutes till the egg whites end up being solid.

NUTRITION INFORMATION

Amount per serving (1 serving) — Calories: 224, Fat: 15g, Saturated Fat: 5g, Cholesterol: 47mg, Potassium: 731mg, Carbohydrates: 14g, Fiber: 5g, Sugar: 7g, Protein: 12G, Vitamin A: 256%, Vitamin C: 4%, Calcium: 275%, Iron: 1%

Pan-Fried Tuscan Chicken Pasta

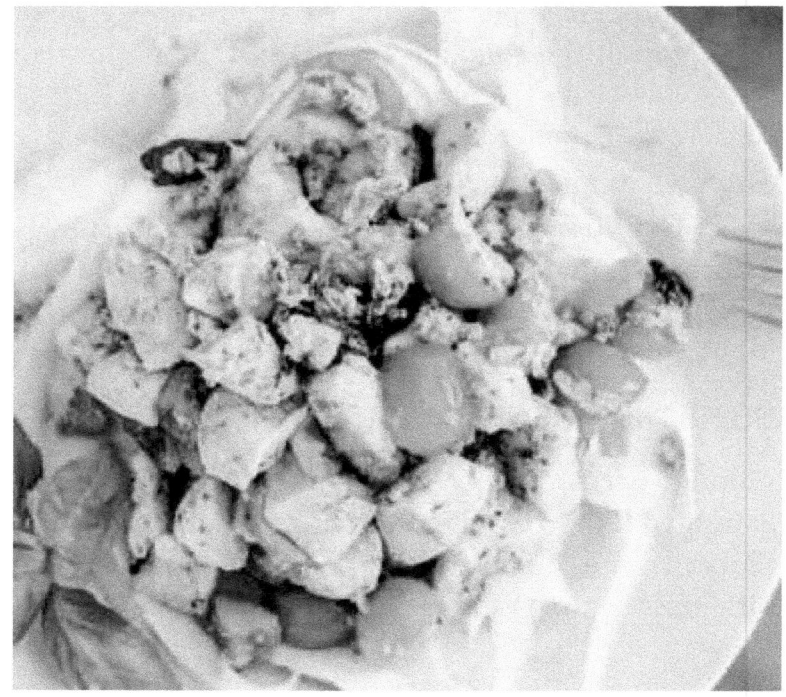

The Chicken is prepared swiftly; it keeps all its taste and doesn't dry out. Also, including basil and tomato, to this pasta recipe, is a fantastic suggestion. Basil is easy to prepare in the pots, so you could have a resource of quality to include in soups and also sauces at any time.

Appreciate this delicious Paleo and Ketogenic Tuscan Chicken pasta without gluten or grains. This recipe makes use of zucchini noodles as the pasta, yet you can likewise use various kinds of Paleo pasta.

This is a straightforward, fast supper to prepare using very easy to discover components like Italian seasoning, eggs, tomatoes, and chicken bust. Make this Tuscan chicken pasta meal on days when you do not have much time to prepare.

Ingredients

- 2 chicken breasts, diced
- 2 little egg, blended
- 1/4 tsp salt
- Dash of black pepper
- 2 tsp garlic powder
- 2 teaspoon Italian flavoring
- 14 cherry tomatoes, cut into quarters
- 30 basil leaves
- Olive oil or avocado oil to prepare in
- Extra salt and pepper to taste
- 1 zucchini, peeled off and become shreds or hairs for the pasta

Steps

- Dice the Chicken bust into tiny cubes. This makes them prepare much faster as well as soak up more of the herbs and also flavors.
- Make the egg sauce for the Chicken pieces making use of eggs, salt, pepper, garlic powder, and also Italian spices. Blend in a bowl.
- Add the diced Chicken to the blended egg mix and coat the chicken pieces thoroughly.
- Prepare the cherry tomatoes by cutting them into quarters, as well as choose 30 fresh basil leaves.

- Add the olive oil or avocado oil to a frying pan and sauté the chicken items with the egg blend. Sauté on a tool heat till the chicken pieces are prepared.
- When the Chicken pieces are prepared, add in the tomatoes and also basil leaves. If you have time, add in 3 cloves of garlic minced for extra taste. Include added salt and pepper to preference.
- While the chicken is cooking, peel zucchini and also use the shredding add-on of a mixer or else a potato peeler to develop shreds or long hairs from the zucchini to ensure that it resembles noodles.
- Split the zucchini noodles in between 2 plates and also put fifty percent of the Chicken sauté on top of each plate of pasta. Garnish with added fresh basil leaves if you want.

NOTES

All dietary data are approximated as well as based on per serving quantities.

NOURISHMENT

Calories: 540 Sugar: 4 g Fat: 36 g Carbohydrates: 7 g Fiber: 2 g Protein: 45 g.

Chicken Noodle Soup

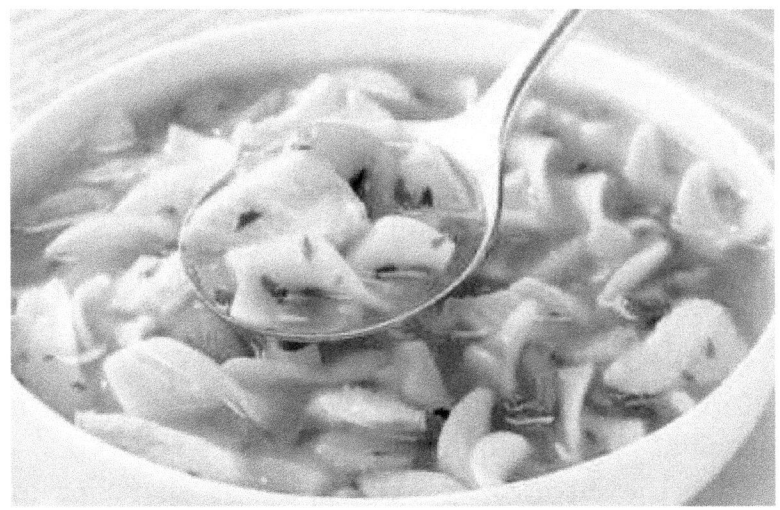

This is a perfect dish to motivate the young ones to eat more veggies. They do not even think about the 'noodles' as vegetables! You can use a potato peeler to develop thin strips or train yourself to use a spiralizer.

Ingredients

- 3 cups chicken brew (use this recipe or get this) (approx. 720ml).
- 1 chicken bust cut right into small portions (approx. 240g or 0.5 pounds).
- 2 tablespoons avocado oil.
- 1 stalk of celery, sliced (approx. 57g).
- 1 green onion, sliced (approx. 10g).
- 1/4 cup cilantro, finely sliced (approx. 15g).

- 1 zucchini, peeled (approx. 106g).
- Salt to taste.

Steps.

- Dice the chicken bust.
- Add the avocado oil right into a pan and sauté the diced chicken in there until cooked.
- Include chicken broth to the same saucepan as well as simmer.
- Cut the celery and add it in the pan.
- Cut the environment-friendly onions as well as include it right into the saucepan.
- Slice the cilantro as well as put it apart for the moment.
- To Produce zucchini noodles, I made use of a potato peeler to produce long strands; however, other options consist of using a spiralizer or a food mill with the shredding accessory.
- Add zucchini noodles as well as cilantro to the pot.
- Boil for a few more minutes, add salt to taste, as well as offer immediately.

NOTES.

All nutritional data are estimated and also based on per serving quantities.

NUTRITION.

Calories: 310 Sugar: 3 g Fat: 16 g Carbohydrates: 6 g Fiber: 2 g Protein: 34 g.

Thai Chicken Pad See Ew

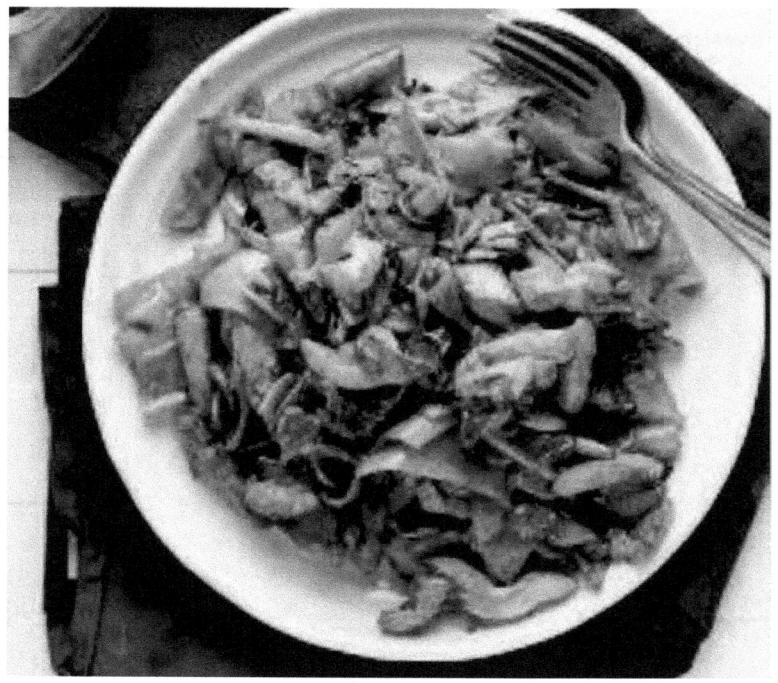

Noodle dishes are few out of the tasty meals, but many noodles simply aren't great for a keto diet; here's where cucumber can be found in. Make use of a Spiralizer or shredder to develop cucumber strips, which are an excellent substitute for rice noodles. This Pad See Ew is very healthy and with balanced goodies, containing protein, vitamins C, K, folic acid, and also anti- inflammatories.

Pad see ew (AKA chicken and also broccoli stir-fried with flat rice noodles) is among my favored Thai dishes, and it's on the menu at most Thai restaurants.

Ingredients

- 1 chicken breast (0.5 lb. or 250 g), cut into tiny, thin pieces
- 1/4 cup (0.6 oz. or 17 g) green onion, diced (scallions).
- 1 cup (4 oz. or 115 g) broccoli florets, broken into tiny florets.
- 1 teaspoon fresh grated ginger.
- 1 tablespoon (15 ml) tamari sauce (use coconut aminos for AIP).
- 2 garlic cloves, minced.
- 1 tablespoon cilantro, finely chopped.
- 1 tablespoon (15 ml) coconut oil to cook in.
- 1 cucumber, peeled into long noodles utilizing a potato peeler.
- Salt to taste.

Steps

- Break the broccoli up into tiny florets.
- Cut the chicken breast right into tiny, thin pieces.
- Grate the ginger, dice the garlic, cut up the environment-friendly onions, as well as cut up the cilantro.
- Place the coconut oil into a sauté pan.
- Add in the chicken the green onions and also sauté.
- Add in the broccoli, ginger, as well as tamari sauce, and then put a lid over the sauté pan, allow let the broccoli chef on medium heat up until it's tender to your preference (approx. 5-10 mins).

- Use a potato peeler to develop strands of long cucumber noodles.
- Split the cucumber noodles between 2 plates.
- Add to the sauté frying pan the minced garlic, cilantro, as well as salt to preference. Separate and serve in addition to the cucumber noodles.

Guidelines.

- Add one tablespoon of coconut oil right into a huge sauté frying pan and also sauté the chicken breast with onions in it.
- Add the broccoli, ginger, and tamari sauce. Place a lid over the pan and allow the broccoli chef on medium warmth till it's tender to your liking (approx. 5-10 minutes). Stir on a regular basis.
- At the same time, peel off the cucumber and later create the cucumber noodles by utilizing a potato peeler to peel the cucumber right into long, vast hairs. Divide the cucumber noodles in between two plates.
- Contribute to the sauté frying pan, the minced garlic, cilantro, as well as salt to preference. Offer on top of the cucumber noodles.

Nourishment Information.

We are serving size: 1 serving-- Calories: 154 Fat: 8 g. Carbohydrates: 11 g. Protein: 11 g.

Paleo Creamy Tomato Pasta

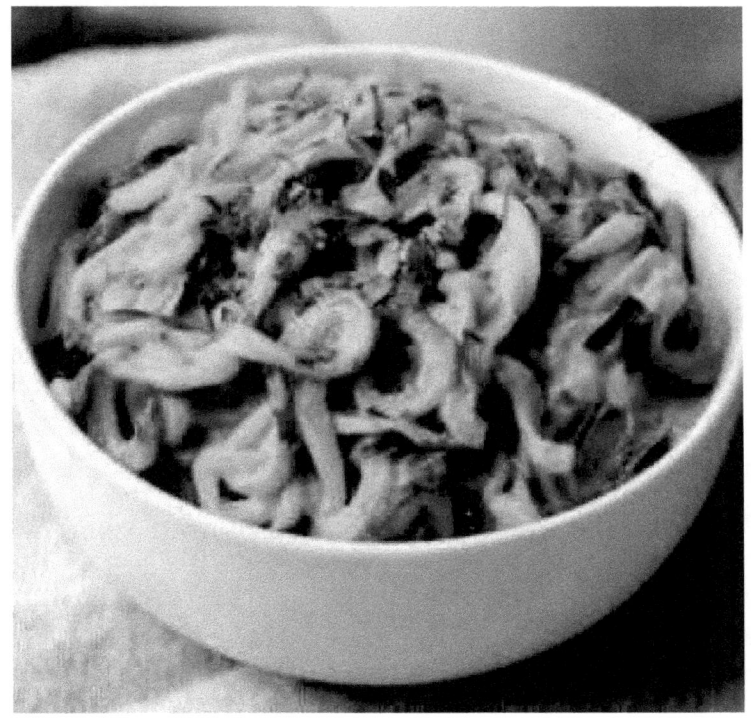

This is a fast and very easy recipe, which is excellent for a quick dish after a busy day. It can also be made reasonably cheap, so it is an excellent meal for pupils! The abundant tastes of tomato and even fragrant basil are so enticing and make this meal preference amazing. If you do not have a spiralizer, you can just shred the zucchini in a food mill or using a grater.

There are lots of various methods to produce Paleo pasta-- from shirataki noodles to cucumber noodles, to spiralized zucchini, to fantastic potato noodles, to also using Paleo flours to present noodles of your very own.

Add fresh tomatoes to this dish to be tastier, and to add in some healthy and balanced fats, and I included coconut milk into the tomato sauce. It merely takes 25 mins from beginning to end.

Ingredients

- 2 chicken breasts, cubed
- 2 tablespoons ghee or coconut oil to prepare in
- 1 can diced tomatoes (14 oz or 400g).
- 1/2 cup basil, sliced.
- 1/4 cup coconut milk.
- 6 cloves garlic, minced.
- Salt to taste.
- 1 zucchini, shredded or spiralized (for the pasta) or pasta squash.

Steps.

- Sauté the diced chicken in the ghee or coconut oil up until cooked as well as slightly browned.
- Add the container of diced tomatoes as well as salt to taste. Place on a simmer as well as prepare the liquid down.
- In the meantime, prepare the pasta. If utilizing zucchinis, shred them in the mixer or.
- Use a julienne peeler or a spiralizer. If making use of spaghetti squash, slice it in half, remove the seeds, cover gently with some coconut oil and microwave each half for 7 mins.
- Include the basil, garlic, and also coconut milk to the chicken and cook for a couple of minutes longer.

- Place half of the pasta right into each dish as well as top with the velvety tomato basil chicken.

-

Notes.

All dietary data are approximated as well as based on per serving amounts.

Serving Size: 1 substantial plate Calories: 540 Sugar: 8 g Fat: 27 g Carbohydrates: 15 g Fiber: 4 g Protein: 59 g.

Goulash with Low Carb Pasta

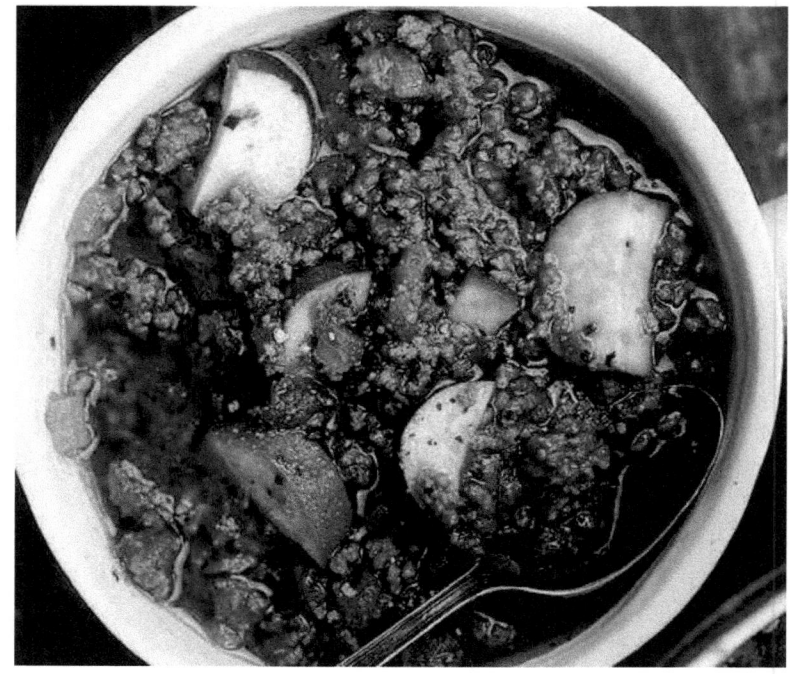

This delicious goulash is full of taste, with sausage, tomato, and a bit of chili powder (which you might opt to overlook if you're not keen on zesty food) and also using shirataki noodles implies this recipe stays low-carb. Very easy to prepare sausage stew recipe with low-carb as well as gluten-free noodles. It's a basic recipe that can be made in about 30 minutes.

The original dish made use of a high fiber pasta product. That product was revealed not to be reduced carbohydrate. So, the meal was upgraded to use ziti shaped shirataki noodles. It's much better with this upgraded as it cut carbohydrate sausage goulash recipe because it's also gluten-free. The noodles utilized initially are made with wheat, so they aren't gluten complimentary.

This reduced carb pasta dish is not only quick and easy to prepare; however, it's tasty also. And, the components can be changed to fit your preference or what you carry hand. While the shirataki noodles are saturating, I like to begin preparing the sausage with onion and garlic until it's browned. In some cases, you can use fresh-cut onions, and various other times, I'll simply include some onion powder. Once the meat is cooked, the remaining components are mixed in. So, the shirataki noodles need to be dried before this step. Then, the mix is covered as well as simmered for about 20 mins and mixed sometimes.

The ziti style noodles are perfect for this low carbohydrate sausage goulash. I used to make use of macaroni noodles back in my high carb days. The ziti Miracle noodles are the ideal low carbohydrate substitute for macaroni.

Ingredients

- 1 7 ounce package shirataki ziti noodles
- 1/2 tsp onion powder
- 2 cloves garlic minced
- 1 pound mass sausage
- 14.5 ounce tinned diced tomatoes
- 1/4 cup chopped celery
- 1 packet stevia
- 1 teaspoon salt
- 1 teaspoon chili powder

Steps

- Drain shirataki noodles, soak in water for 5 mins, drain once again, then stir fry in a dry pan till noodle feel like they are sticking to the pan.
- Prepare sausage with onion powder and also garlic until brown.
- Drain pipes off fat as needed.
- Include the remaining ingredients.
- Simmer covered for about 20 minutes, mixing often.

Meatball Zoodle Soup

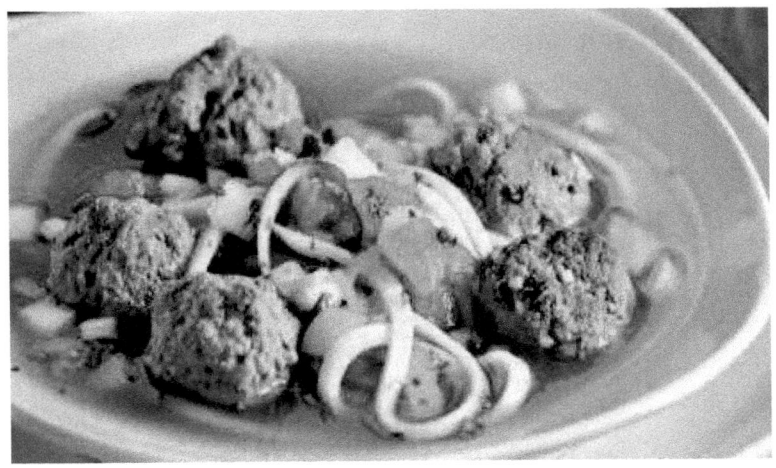

This is another soup-based dish that is wonderful, using remaining vegetables from suppers. To obtain a good structure for your meatballs, you can add some ground pork in with the beef. If you don't have a spiralizer, you can purchase zoodles for this dish. Calories: 129, Carbohydrates: 3g, Fat: 6 g and Protein: 15 g.

Ingredients.

- 32 oz beef supply.
- 1 tool zucchini, Spiraled.
- 2 ribs celery, chopped.
- 1 tiny onion, diced.
- 1 carrot, cut.
- 1 tool tomato, diced.
- 1 1/2 tsp garlic salt.
- 1 1/2 pound ground beef.

- 1/2 cup Parmesan cheese, shredded.
- 6 cloves garlic, minced.
- 1 large egg.
- 4 tbsp fresh parsley, sliced.
- 1 1/2 tsp sea salt.
- 1 1/2 tsp onion powder.
- 1 tsp Italian flavoring.
- 1 tsp dried oregano.
- 1/2 tsp black pepper.

Steps.

- Heat slow-moving cooker on the reduced setting.
- To the sluggish stove, add beef stock, zucchini, celery, onion, carrot, tomato, as well as garlic salt, then cover it.
- In a big mixing dish, mix hamburger, Parmesan, garlic, egg, parsley, sea salt, onion powder, oregano, Italian seasoning, as well as pepper.
- Mix till all ingredients are well integrated—kind right into around 30 meatballs.
- Heat olive oil in a huge skillet over medium-high heat. As soon as the pan is warm, add meatballs and brown on all sides.
- Add meatballs to slow down cooker, cover, and also cook for 6 hrs.

Zucchini Pasta with Bacon Pesto

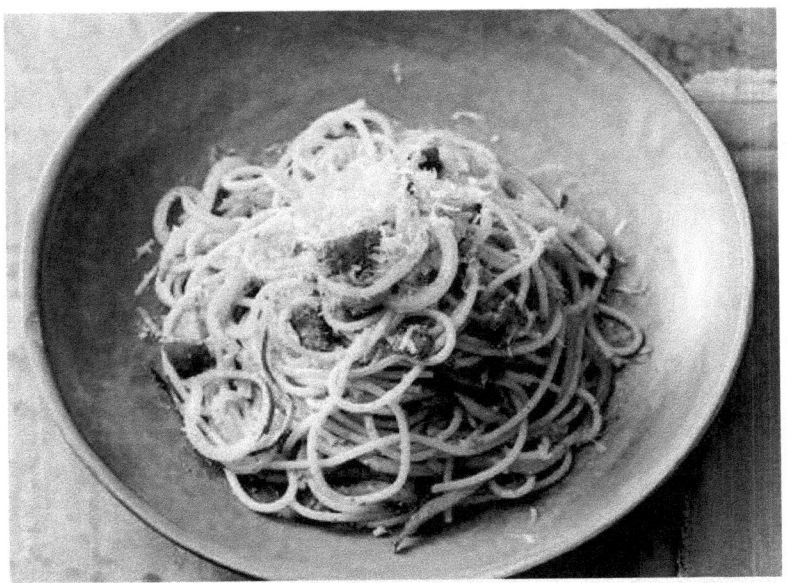

Making bacon from pesto is something you need to attempt at least when bacon is cooked and form a crisp while it cools down, it can be mixed into a yummy, crunchy pesto when blended with oil. The pesto is an excellent sauce for zoodles or any other veggie pasta you fancy making. Mix in a little even more oil, and you've got yourself an intriguing salad dressing, not to mention a functional enhancement to your recipe.

Ingredients

- 10 rashers smoked bacon
- 2 cloves garlic, diced
- 1/4 cup mint leaves, loaded

- 1/2 cup basil leaves, packed
- 3/4 cup flat-leaf parsley, loaded
- 3/4 cup olive oil
- 3 big zucchini
- Fine sea salt to taste

Instructions

- Preheat the griddle.
- Lay the bacon rashers on a big baking tray and also broil for 10 to 12 mins until crispy.
- Transfer to a large plate lined with absorptive kitchen area paper and enable it to cool and solidify.
- Pour the fat into a small container.
- When the bacon is crunchy, break rashers into large pieces as well as take into a food processor, together with the remaining pesto components. Blitz up until you have an instead loosened paste with small grain-sized bacon portions for appearance.
- At the same time, prepare the zucchini noodles. Cut off each zucchini and peel the skin if you desire (I didn't). Making use of a spiralizer or a julienne peeler, make "pasta" from each one, clipping midway to stop them being also long.
- Heat a tbsp of the reserved bacon fat in a vast sauté frying pan (scheduling any more for another usage), include the zucchini, and cook for around 5 mins on a low-medium warm-up until tender.
- Put noodles into a bowl-shaped sieve and drain well.
- Currently, turn off the warm, wipe out the sauté frying pan with cooking area paper as well as return the zucchini to the pan. Add the pesto and also blend well, so the noodles are equally covered.

- Have a fast taste and add salt if needed, though you may find your bacon makes it salted sufficient.
- Offer quickly.

Sun-Dried Tomato Pesto and Sausage Pasta

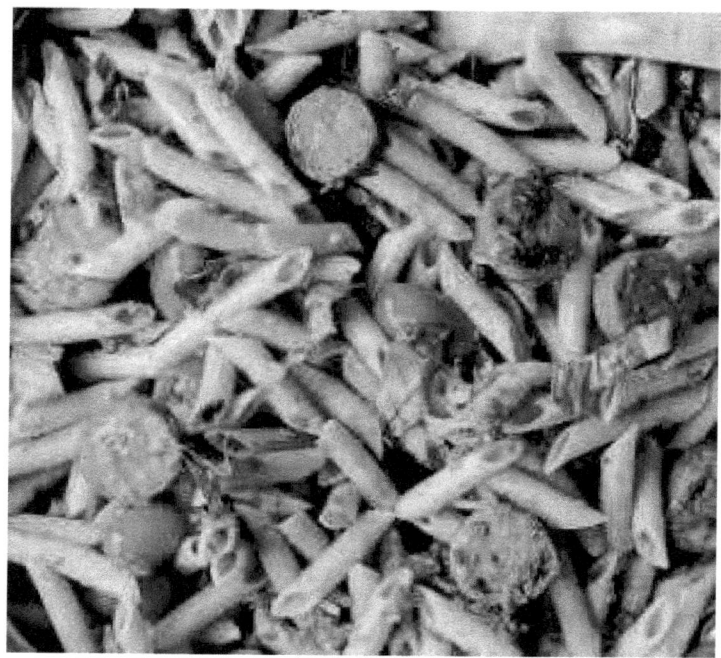

One of the best benefits of making use of zucchini to make your spaghetti is that it is ready much quicker than pasta. The pesto in this recipe uses tomatoes, parsley as well as pine nuts to make a delicious sauce for any recipe, however it functions specifically well with the sausage.

Ingredients

- 4-5 medium-sized zucchini (or sub pasta of selection).
- 1 lb. Sweet Italian sausage, cases removed.
- 1 onion, diced.

- 1 tbsp olive oil.
- 1 tablespoon minced garlic.

For the Pesto.

- 1-8.5 ounce container sun-dried tomatoes in oil.
- 1/4 cup reserved oil from sun-dried tomatoes.
- 1 cup of fresh basil leaves.
- 1/4 cup of fresh parsley.
- 1/2 cup pine nuts.
- 2 tsp. Lemon juice.
- 1-15-oz can diced tomatoes, drained.
- 1/2 tsp oregano.
- 1/2 tsp garlic powder.
- Salt and pepper to taste.
- Garnish.
- Sliced fresh basil and also parsley.

Ingredients.

- Spiralize your zucchini and also set aside in a huge pot.
- In a large frying pan, cook sausage, onion, and also garlic till sausage is browned and well prepared.
- Drain your sun-dried tomatoes, booking 1/4 cup of oil.
- In a food mill, incorporate sun-dried tomatoes, basil, parsley, ache nuts, and 1/4 cup reserved oil. Refine up until the herbs, tomatoes, and also nuts have broken up well. Add the remaining to be ingredients and also procedure up until thick as well as somewhat velvety.
- Add pesto sauce to the frying pan with the sausage and also mix periodically, until warmed.

- Cook zucchini noodles on tool heat as well as mix sometimes, till softened, concerning 5-7 minutes. Drain pipes excess water.
- Plate zucchini noodles, top with pesto sausage sauce, and add fresh herbs.

Autoimmune Paleo Spaghetti Squash Chicken Pasta

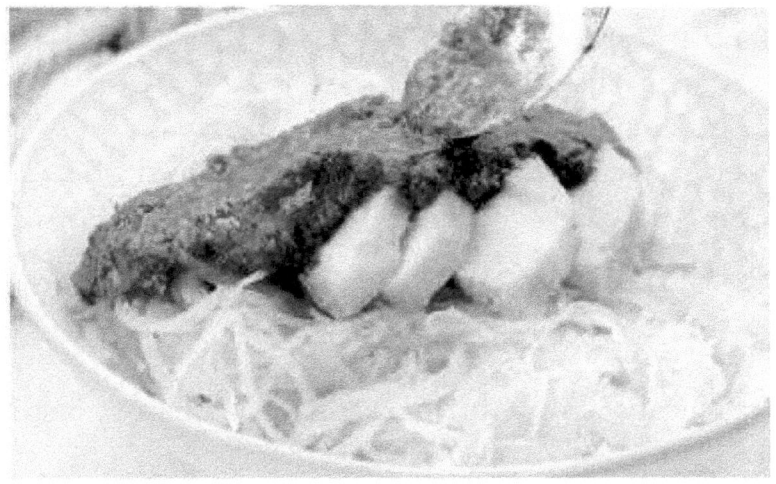

The pasta in this dish is, in fact, nut-free, which is best for any person that suffers from nut allergy reaction. Chicken is the excellent enhancement to a pesto based dish, precisely when it is seasoned with sweet basil and sharp arugula. Pasta squash is made use of to change pasta in this dish as well as is made with baked squash, which offers it an authentic al-dente texture.

Use either chicken thighs or breasts for this dish. Basil & arugula produce the base for the creamy pesto. Basil offers its sweet, floral tones, arugula, includes more of bite. The flavor of your olive oil will surely radiate through.

Ingredients

- 1 tool spaghetti squash.

- 1 lb. Boneless skinless chicken breast or upper legs.
- 1 tbsp coconut oil (or various other cooking fat).
- 1 cup basil.
- 1 cup arugula.
- 1/2 cup olive oil.
- one lemon juice.
- 1 clove of garlic, peeled off and also minced.
- Sea salt to taste.

Steps.

- Preheat the oven to 400 F, and also line two baking sheets with parchment paper.
- Cook the spaghetti squash as advised.
- While the pasta squash is baking, add the chicken bust to the various other baking sheets. Add the coconut oil to the hen and period with salt.
- Cook in the oven for 20-25 mins or up until a thermostat checks out 160 F.
- When the pasta squash and also chicken are done, scoop the spaghetti squash right into a bowl, top with sliced chicken.
- For the pesto, add the basil, arugula, olive oil, lemon juice, garlic, and salt to a high-speed blender and also blend till smooth.
- Top the pasta squash and also chicken with pesto, to enjoy! Store any leftover pesto in the refrigerator for 2-3 days.

AIP Paleo Spaghetti with Meat Sauce

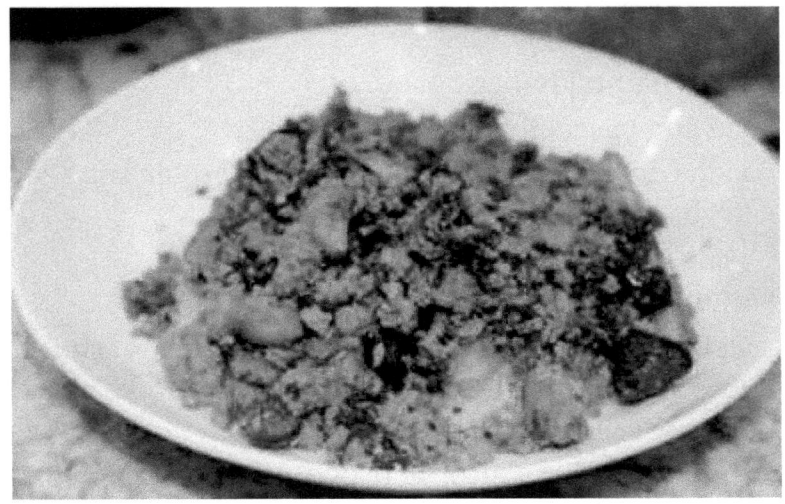

This meaty-sauced pastas meal is flavored with black olives, garlic, spinach, and also mushrooms. Using squash as spaghetti is an excellent means to replace pasta in this meal. Nonetheless, you can select zoodles if it is your favorite. Sprinkle with a significant portion of Nutritional Yeast for a much more tacky taste! Coconut milk makes the sauce more velvety like Alfredo. If you haven't tried it, you should. It's appetizing!

Ingredients

- One portion of pasta squash cooked & shredded or my new favorite AIP compliant noodle (glass noodles).
- 2 pounds natural turf fed hamburger.
- 1 Tbs. Olive oil.

- 1 1/2 oz cut onions.
- 5-6 cloves of minced fresh garlic or dehydrated minced garlic.
- Sea salt to preference.
- 1 Tbs natural Italian spices.
- 1/2 cup black olives.
- 1 sm container of fresh sliced up mushrooms or 1 can of natural sliced mushrooms.
- 1 bag of natural baby spinach.
- Dietary yeast optional (for cheesy taste).
- Optional-- For AIP add 1-2 containers of full-fat coconut milk (for creamier more Alfredo-like sauce), I like to include 2 cans.
- Optional-- For Paleo, add one container of natural diced tomatoes or your favorite marinara sauce.

Steps

- Sauté onions & garlic on a medium heat using olive oil, until they become tender & translucent.
- Add hamburger, sea salt & cook until brown.
- Add Italian flavoring, olives & mushrooms & cook until mushrooms are done.
- If you are adding either coconut milk or tomatoes, add them now.
- Let simmer for about 15-20 minutes.
- Add spinach.
- Sprinkle with Nutritional Yeast.
- Serve over spaghetti squash or glass noodles.

Tip- Make sure you add enough sea salt & garlic powder to the pasta squash.

Notes.

Make sure you add enough sea salt & garlic to the pasta squash, or it could be a little as well fantastic.

Bacon Herb Spaghetti Squash "Pasta" Salad

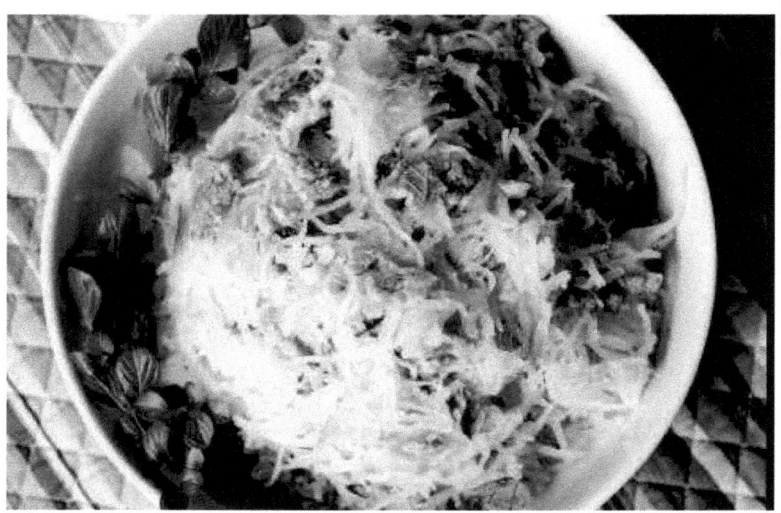

Not all pasta meals need to be served hot; this spaghetti squash dish is fresh, best for warm summertime day when you're starving, just opt for this easy salad. Make a big batch as well as pop it in the refrigerator prepared for the whole house's lunch to go tomorrow!

This AIP "pasta" salad tastes wonderful either if it is cooled or warmed suitable for any outing or work.

Ingredients.

- 1 spaghetti squash.
- 3 tbsp bacon oil or lard.
- 1/2 tsp raw salt.
- 1/2 tsp dried out thyme.
- 1/4 tsp black pepper (omit if desired).

- 1/2 tsp celery salt or dried out marjoram for AIP.
- 1/4 tsp ground dried out the sage.
- 1/2 cup fresh oregano, chopped.
- 3/4 to 1 cup sliced cooked bacon (if you can get smoked hog dewlaps, those are also better!).
-

Steps.

- Preheat oven to 350F.
- Slice spaghetti squash in half lengthwise using a sharp blade. Dig as well as dispose of seeds.
- Separate bacon grease into half and place it in the scooped out holes. Split dry flavorings in half and spread uniformly over the cut fifty percent.
- Place squash halves reduced side up in a glass recipe as well as include 1/4 -1/2-inch water to the bottom of the meal.
- Cover with an ovenproof cover or foil and bake for about 30-40 mins, depending on just how large your own is. If you don't have pre-cooked bacon, lay slices in a solitary layer on a cookie sheet with a rim and bake while the squash is cooking. Depending on how thick the bacon is, it will probably require you to cook for 10-20 mins.
- Once it is done to your liking, get rid of, allow trendy, then cut coarsely.
- When the spaghetti squash is done, get rid of the oven. Once it is cool enough to take care of, remove the squash shreds using two forks and also place in a big bowl.

- Mix in the chopped fresh oregano and bacon. Cover and cool in the fridge for several hrs until cooled down throughout.
- Optional: Add numerous ounces of leftover shredded chicken (or other meat) to make it a full dish for a picnic or jam-packed lunch.
- Served chilled. However, you can take it when it is hot if that is fine with you. Simply reheat in the stove for some mins till warmed enough. Season with salt or pepper!

Zucchini Noodle Bolognese

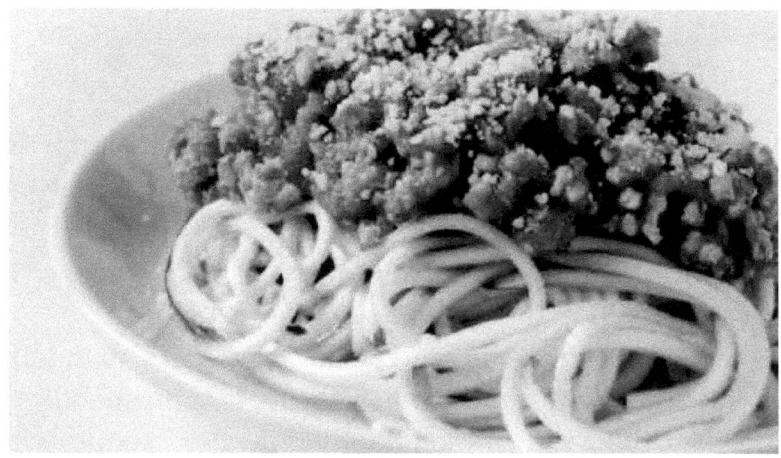

Spaghetti Bolognese is among those conventional Italian pasta meals, which will bring warm memories for many, but you can make a much healthier, Keto-friendly version of this in your home. Instead of using hamburger, Italian sausage gives a slightly various taste to this classic.

Ingredients

- 6 medium zucchini
- 1/2 pound light Italian sausage (bulk or coverings removed).
- 1 tablespoon avocado oil (or chosen cooking oil).
- 1/8 cup water.
- 1 orange bell pepper, seeded and also diced.
- 6 ramps (or 1 small diced onion + 2-3 cloves of garlic).
- 1 extra pound pearl or roma tomatoes.

- Sea salt.
- Black pepper.

Steps

- Clean ramps. Remove and discard roots. Chop the fallen leaves off over the pink stems and. DO NOT discard the leaves
- Chop them up very well, keep 2 tablespoons to garnish. Chop the ramps.
- Peel zucchini. Spiralize zucchini or use a mandolin and also pieces zucchini to form "lengthy noodles." Place them in a colander and also spray with concerning a teaspoon of sea salt.
- Heat oil in a frying pan on medium-high heat. Place cut ramps and also leaves in the skillet in addition to the sausage, bell pepper, salt, and pepper to taste. Cook for 5 minutes up until sausage is practically cooked through.
- Slice tomatoes in half and also place level side down on sausage blend.
- Add water to the skillet, cover and reduce the heat—steam for 15 mins.
- Remove the lid and cook for another 10 minutes while sauce thickens, chopping the tomatoes with the side of your mixing spoon.
- Boil water in a medium pot. Cook zucchini for 3-4 mins until tender. Drain pipes.
- Serve your noodles. Garnish with chopped ramp leaves.

Garlic Shrimp Zucchini Pasta.

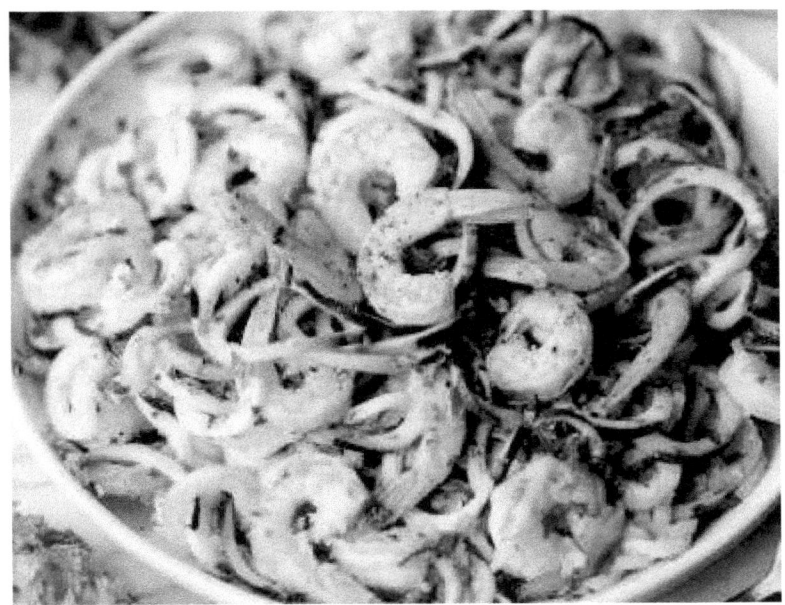

Ingredients

- 4 large zucchini (about 2 extra pounds).
- 2 tsp Salt (to salt the zucchini).
- 1/3 cup bacon oil (crispy bits make it even much better).
- 1/4 cup chopped fresh basil.
- 2 large garlic cloves, squashed.
- 1/2 cup sliced Walnuts (optional, leave out for AIP).

Instructions

- Cut the ends off of your to fit your spiralizer.

- Run your zucchini through your spiralizer. In a large pan, sauté your zucchini noodles with your olive oil, onion, and keep seasonings up until onion and zucchini are soft. Add your shrimp up until warmed and serve.
- This dish features zucchini as a mock noodle, which has a sweet flavor for Italian-inspired meals.
- Omit the walnuts to make this autoimmune recipe protocol-friendly. This recipe makes sufficient for 3- 4 hearty side dish portions.
- Alternately, you might include some barbequed steak, prawns, or chicken. Serves 3-4.

Low Carb Keto Noodles Options

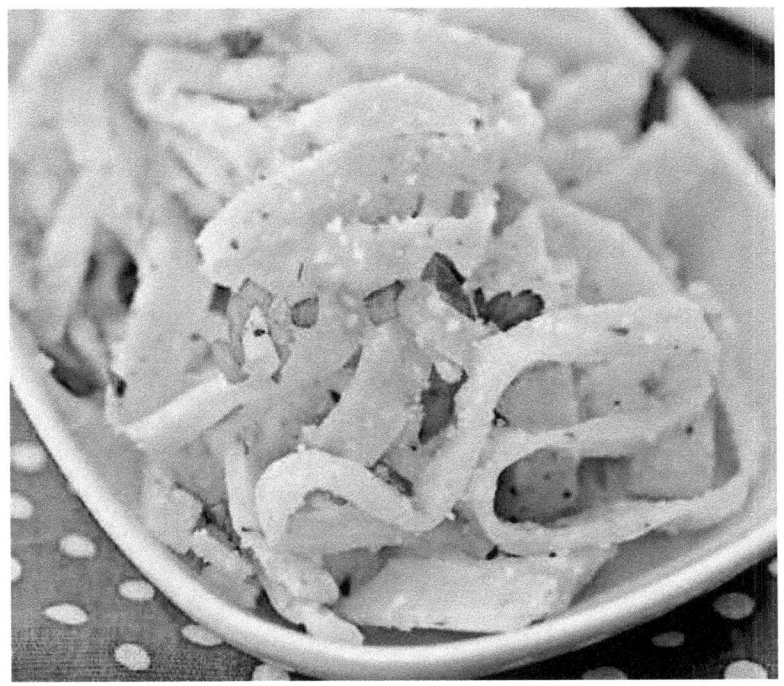

Low carbohydrate keto cabbage noodles are always a family fave.

Ingredients

- 1 extra pound cabbage, cored and also cut into strips
- 1/4 cup onions, chopped very finely (1 oz).
- 2 cloves garlic, sliced.
- 2 tablespoon butter or oil.
- Salt and pepper to preference.

Instructions.

- Cut the cabbage quarterly by cutting out the central part it into strips. Finely slice the onions and cut the garlic.
- Heat a pan over a medium temperature. When it is hot, add the butter or oil and swirl to coat the frying pan.
- Add the cabbage, onion and also garlic and sauté up until the cabbage hurts - concerning 10 minutes.
- Salt and pepper to taste.

Percent Daily Values are based upon a 2000 calorie diet plan.

Keto Creamy Avocado Pasta with Shirataki

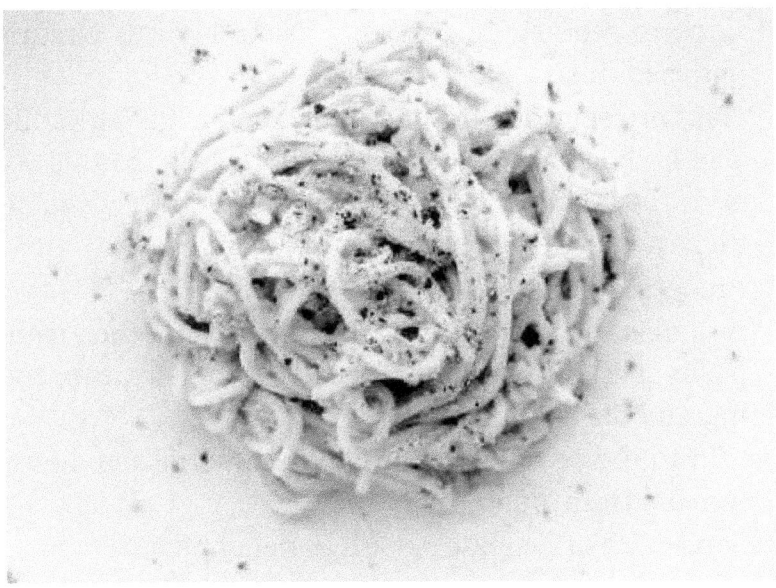

Ingredients.

- 1 packet of shirataki noodles.
- 1 avocado ripe.
- 1/4 cup whipping cream.
- 1 tsp dried out basil.
- 1 tsp black pepper.
- 1 tsp salt.

Instructions.

- Prepare the shirataki.
- Drain the shirataki noodles in a colander to remove the liquid they come packaged. Wash thoroughly

under running water. If the noodles are still long, cut into much shorter items with scissors.

- Steam some water and also cook the shirataki for 1- 2 mins to remove any sticking around scent. Drain it and also rinse again.
- Heat a clean, dry fry pan and pour in the shirataki. The noodles have vast amounts of water, so this will assist dry them. Cook for a minute until they start to make a whistling sound. Remove from heat.
- Prepare the sauce.
- In a dish, mash your avocado and include the cream, basil, salt, and pepper. For a smoother texture, mix ingredients in a mixer.
- Add to the frying pan with your shirataki noodles as well as stir through.
- Serve hot with cheese as well as delight in!

15-Minute Garlic Shrimp Noodles.

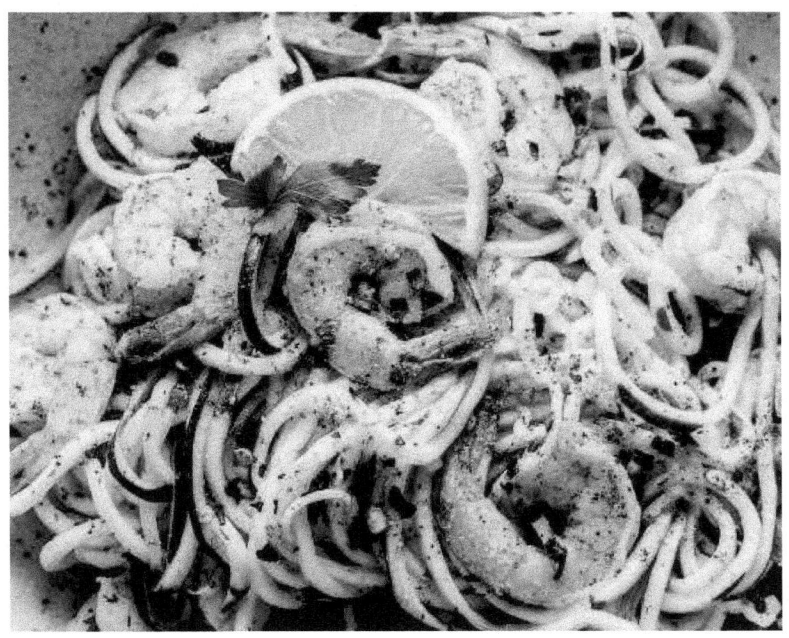

Ingredients.

- 2 medium zucchini.
- 3/4 pounds tool shrimp peeled off & deveined.
- 1 tablespoon olive oil.
- 1 lemon Juice.
- 3-4 cloves garlic minced.
- Red pepper flakes (optional).
- Salt & pepper to preference.
- Cut fresh parsley.

Instructions

- Spiralize the zucchini on the medium setting.
- Add the olive oil as well as lemon juice & passion to a skillet on medium heat. Once the pan is cozy, add the shrimp. Prepare the shrimp for one min per side.
- Include the garlic and red pepper flakes. Cook for an added minute, stirring often.
- Include the zucchini noodles and also stir/toss (e.g., with tongs) continuously for 2-3 minutes until they're a little prepared and heated up.
- Season with salt and pepper, and also sprinkle with the sliced parsley. Offer promptly.

Notes: Calories 276

Calories from Fat 90

Sodium 1339mg 58%

Potassium 686mg 20%

Carbohydrates 9g 3%

Fiber 2G 8%

Sugar 5g 6%

Protein 38g 76%

Garlic Gnocchi

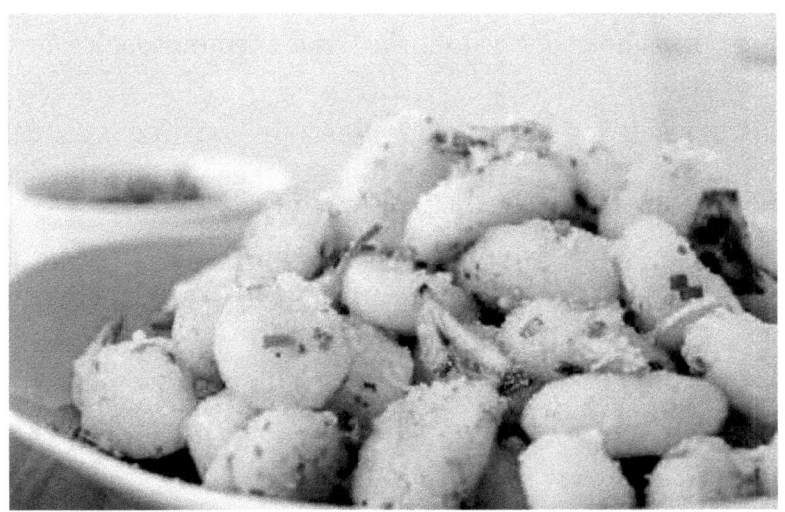

Ingredients.

- 2 cups shredded Mozzarella (Low-Moisture Part-Skim this is a MUST-- or else it will certainly break down when boiled!).
- 3 egg yolks.
- 1 tsp granulated garlic.
- Butter & olive oil for sautéing.

Ingredients:

- Place cheese and garlic in a risk-free microwave bowl and combine. Melt cheese in the microwave for about 1 to 1 1/2 minutes.
- Fold up in one egg yolk at a time until a uniform dough forms. This actually takes a little effort!

- Portion dough into four spheres.
- Chill in the refrigerator for at least 10 mins.
- Lightly grease a Silpat or parchment (use your hands to prevent it from sticking!) and turn out each round into a 14-15 " log.
- Cut each log into one " item. (If you like, you can push the tip of a fork onto each piece to obtain that "gnocchi" look, but it's not necessary).
- In a huge pot, produce a half gallon of salted water to a simmer. Place all the gnocchi into the bowl and cook up until they float, concerning 2-3 minutes.
- Warm a big non-stick pan on medium-high heat. Add a tablespoon of butter and a tablespoon of oil to the frying pan.
- Include gnocchi as well as sauté each side for concerning 1-2 minutes, until gold brownish.
- Season with salt and pepper and offer!

Keto Carbonara Pasta.

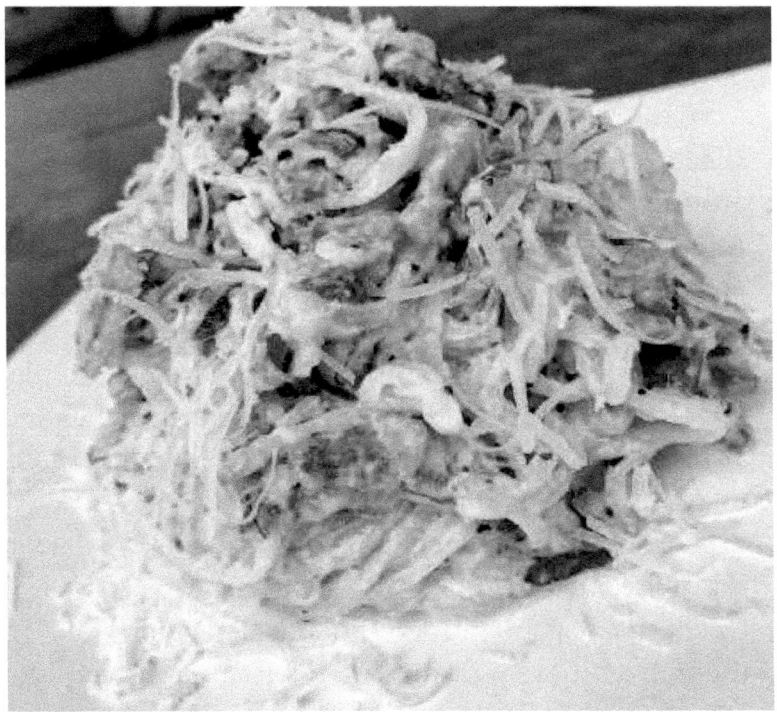

Carbonara pasta is such a straightforward keto recipe, super velvety, and such a simple household dinner as a substitute for regular pasta or for family members.

Ingredients

- 60 g Chicken Breast 2 oz.
- 150 g bacon 5 oz.
- 1 Cup heavy whipping cream, Thicken Cream.
- 1 Large Egg Yolk.
- 2 Tbsp Parmesan cheese.
- 1 Packet Miracle Noodles.

Steps.

- Dice the bacon, and cook in a frying pan until the outside changes color, but not go crispy. Remove from the pan.
- Dice the chicken and also do the same—Cook for around 5 minutes. Remove from the pan.
- In a little bowl, blend the egg yolk and also the parmesan cheese together up until it develops a paste.
- In the previous fry pan on tool heat, add 1/2 the total quantity of cream, and also mix the parmesan as well as egg mixture into the cream. This will require some mixing.
- Finally, add the cream and the chicken and bacon. Continue stirring.
- Open the bag of miracle noodles, and also dry fry them in a different frying pan for 10 mins.
- Mix the proper noodles right into the sauce and serve.

Fresh Egg Pasta.

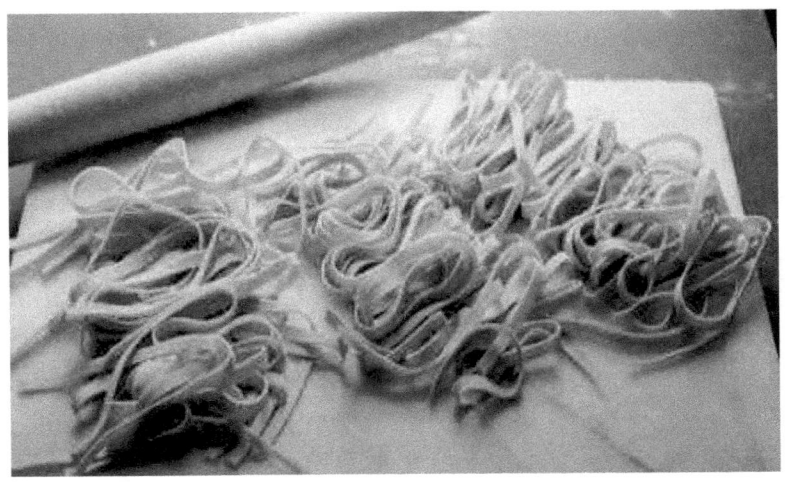

Ingredients.

FOR THE KETO PASTA DOUGH.

- 96 g almond flour.
- 24 g coconut flour.
- 2 teaspoons xanthan gum.
- 1/4 teaspoon kosher salt.
- 2 tsp. Apple cider vinegar.
- 1 egg lightly defeated.
- 2-4 teaspoons water as required.
- 56 g grass-fed saltless butter as needed.
- 2 tablespoons extra virgin olive oil.
- 4 cloves garlic slivered, optional (however extremely suggested!).

Steps.

FOR THE KETO PASTA DOUGH.

- Add almond flour, coconut flour, xanthan gum tissue, and salt to the food grinder.
- Keep in mind: you can additionally blend them in a big dish and use your hand or stand mixer for the adhering to actions.
- Mesh apple cider vinegar with the mixer running. Once it has circulated uniformly, pour in the egg.
- Add water using a teaspoon, as required, till the dough turns right into a ball. The dough should be firm yet sticky to touch and also without any folds (which means the mixture is completely dry, and you need to include a little bit much more water).
- If no food grinder is at hand, you can likewise do it by hand (it merely takes a bit more time and muscle mass!). Add all the dry components to a big dish as well as whisk up until extensively incorporated.
- Gather vinegar and blend up until extensively distributed.
- Gather egg while blending strongly as well as maintain whisking until the dough comes to be also stiff to mix.
- Using your hands, massaged the dough till thoroughly mixed, adding a tsp of water at once as needed (we make use of 2).
- Wrap dough and also massaged it through the plastic for a couple of minutes. Allow mixture to rest for 30 minutes (and approximately five days) in the fridge.

TO SHAPE IT

For farfalle: turn out the pasta to its thinnest point using a tortilla press in between parchment paper (our fave) or a pasta machine. You can additionally make use of a moving pin, but it'll take a little longer. Cut into roughly 2x1-inch rectangular shapes. And if you're unclear about discussion, use a blade to cut lengthwise and also a pastry cutter to cut widthwise.

For orecchiette: cut dough into four items, turn out into even-sized logs as well as slice off even-sized items. This will undoubtedly make sure evenly-sized pasta. Utilizing your thumb, press each piece versus your contrary hand, developing an impression. Lightly dust with coconut flour as needed. You can either leave them as they are or transform them out.

For cavatelli: cut dough into four pieces, roll out into even-sized logs, and also trim even-sized items. This will undoubtedly make sure evenly-sized pasta. Lightly dust the board and pasta with coconut flour. Place an article on the board as well as utilizing a blade press the dough towards you, angling the knife suggestion upwards as you press, making the pasta curl into form.

Place the shaped pasta in the freezer for 15 minutes (as well as up to a couple of months).

To Cook

- Heat-up butter and oil in a low-temperature pan. Once cozy, include garlic slivers. When the garlic starts to brown, include cooled pasta as well as baste as soon as possible.

- Cook pasta till it merely starts to obtain some color, we discovered this provided one of the most 'al dente' appearance (soft but with a bite). Do not hesitate to make a test with one item.
- Serve immediately with toppings of option.

Notes

Do not hesitate to go on and freeze the pasta, however, and you'll wish to defrost it out slightly before food preparation.

This dish returns approximately 200g of pasta. We computed nourishment realities for a 50g offering (4g net carbs), bearing in mind that this keto pasta is quite a bit much more filling than the typical.

Zucchini Ravioli.

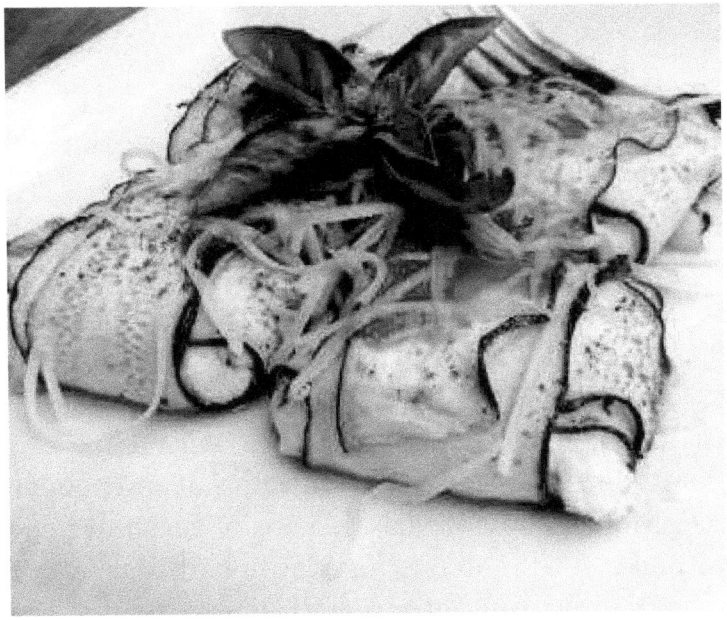

Zucchini noodles can stand in for far more than spaghetti.

Ingredients.

- Extra-virgin olive oil, for baking dish.
- 4 medium zucchini.
- 2 c. ricotta.
- 1/2 c. freshly grated Parmesan, plus a lot more for garnish.
- 1 huge egg, gently beaten.
- 1/4 c. very finely sliced basil, split.
- 1 clove garlic, minced.
- Kosher salt.
- Fresh ground black pepper.

- 2 c. marinara.
- 1/2 c. shredded mozzarella.

Steps.

- Preheat oven to 375 ° and grease a big baking dish with olive oil.
- Make the noodles: Slice two sides of each zucchini lengthwise to develop 2 level sides.
- Making use of a vegetable peeler, slice each zucchini right into slim flat strips, peeling off up until you reach the facility.
- In a tool bowl, combine ricotta, Parmesan, egg, 2 tbsps. Basil, garlic, and season with salt and pepper.
- Assemble the ravioli: Lay 2 strips of zucchini noodles to make sure that they overlap lengthwise. Lay two more noodles on top, perpendicular to the first strips. You should wind up with a "T" form. Bring ends of the strips together to fold over the center, working one side at a time.
- Transform pasta over in the baking dish seam side down. Repeat with remaining zucchini and also filling. Pour marinara around zucchini and also top pasta with mozzarella.
- Cook till zucchini noodles are "al dente" and cheese is melty and has gold on top, within 25 to 30 mins.
- Top with remaining basil and also Parmesan before you serve.

Nutrition (per offering): 220 calories, 17 g protein, 11 g carbs, 2 g fiber, 3 g sugar, 12 g fat, 7 g hydrogenated fat, 500 mg sodium.

Keto Mac & Cheese.

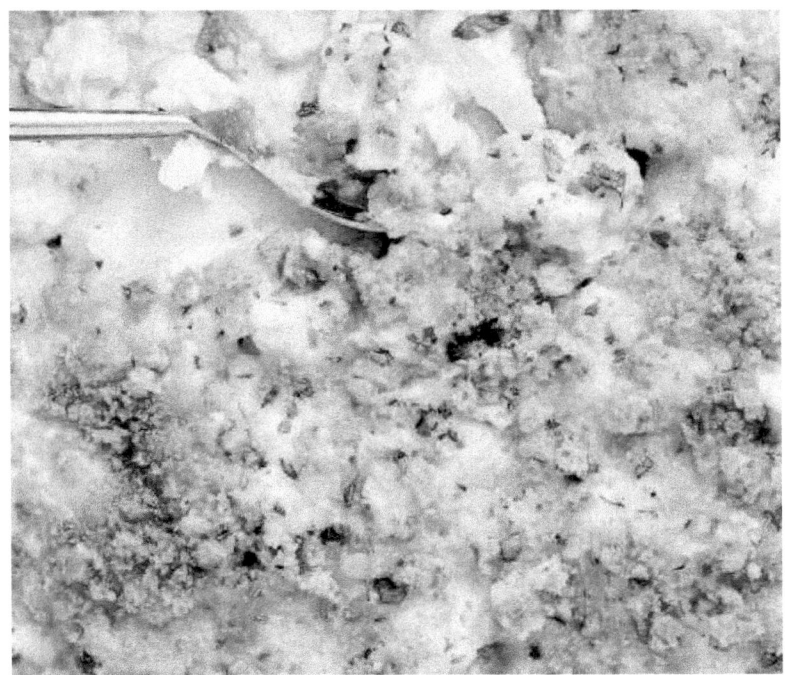

Ingredients

FOR THE MAC & CHEESE.

- Butter, for cooking.
- 2 medium heads cauliflower, cut into florets.
- 2 tablespoon. Extra-virgin olive oil.
- Kosher salt.
- 1 c. heavy cream.
- 6 oz. Cream cheese, cut into cubes.
- 4 c. shredded cheddar.
- 2 c. shredded mozzarella.
- 1 tablespoon hot sauce (optional).

- Fresh ground black pepper.

FOR THE TOPPING.

- 4 oz. Pork rinds, crushed.
- 1/4 c. fresh grated Parmesan.
- 1 tablespoon. Extra-virgin olive oil.
- 2 tablespoon. Freshly sliced parsley, for garnish.
-

Steps.

- Preheat oven to 375 ° and also butter 9"- x-13" baking dish. In a big plate, toss cauliflower with 2 tbsp—oil and season with salt.
- Spread cauliflower onto 2 big baking sheets as well as roast till tender and gently golden, about 40 minutes.
- Meanwhile, in a big pot over medium heat, heat cream. Raise to a simmer, then reduce heat to low and mix in cheeses up until melted. Eliminate from heat, include hot sauce if using and also season with salt and pepper, then layer in roasted cauliflower. Taste and period much more if needed.
- Transfer mixture to prepare the baking meal. In a medium container stir to combine pork rinds, Parmesan, and oil. Sprinkle the mixture in an even layer over cauliflower and cheese.
- Cook up until golden, 15 minutes. If preferred, turn oven to broil to toast topping further, concerning 2 mins.
- Garnish with parsley before serving.

Cauliflower Baked Ziti

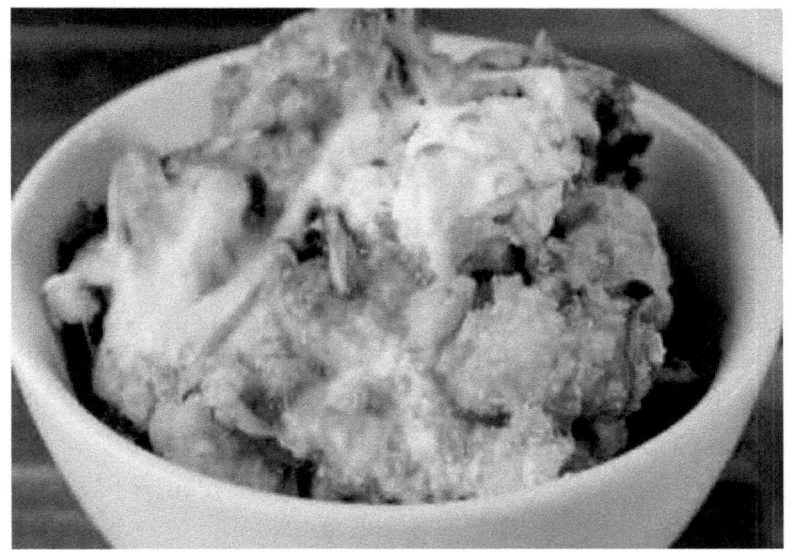

. Ingredients

- 1 tablespoon. Extra-virgin olive oil.
- 1 tool onion, chopped.
- 2 garlic cloves, diced.
- Squeeze red pepper flakes.
- 1 lb. Hamburger.
- Kosher salt.
- Freshly ground black pepper.
- 2 tbsp. Tomato paste.
- 1 tsp. Dried out oregano.
- 1 (28-oz.) can crushed tomatoes.
- 2 tablespoon. Thinly cut basil, plus much more for garnish.

- 1 large head of cauliflower (concerning 3 cups) cut into florets, blanched, and also drained well.
- 1 1/2 c. fresh ricotta.
- 2 c. shredded mozzarella.
- 1/2 c. freshly grated Parmesan.

Steps.

- Preheat oven to 375 °. In a large saucepan over medium heat, warm oil. Add onion and also cook, keep stirring up until onion is soft, about 5 mins.
- Mix in garlic and also red pepper flakes as well as cook for one minute.
- Add meat and season with salt and pepper. Prepare until no longer pink, 6 mins. Drain fat.
- Return pan over tool heat and also add tomato paste and also oregano.
- Cook for 2 mins much more, until slightly dimmed. Add crushed tomatoes and bring sauce to a simmer, reduce heat and cook, occasionally stirring, until slightly lowered and also flavors have combined, 10 to 15 mins. Remove from heat and stir in basil.
- In a big bowl, put the sauce over cauliflower and also mix to combine.
- In a huge cooking container, place half the cauliflower in an even layer. Blob around with half the ricotta, and spray with half the mozzarella as well as Parmesan.
- Add the remainder of the cauliflower in an even layer ahead, and also top with continuing to be cheeses.

- Cook till cheese is melty and golden, 25 minutes. Garnish with basil before serving.

Cacio E Pepe Egg Noodles.

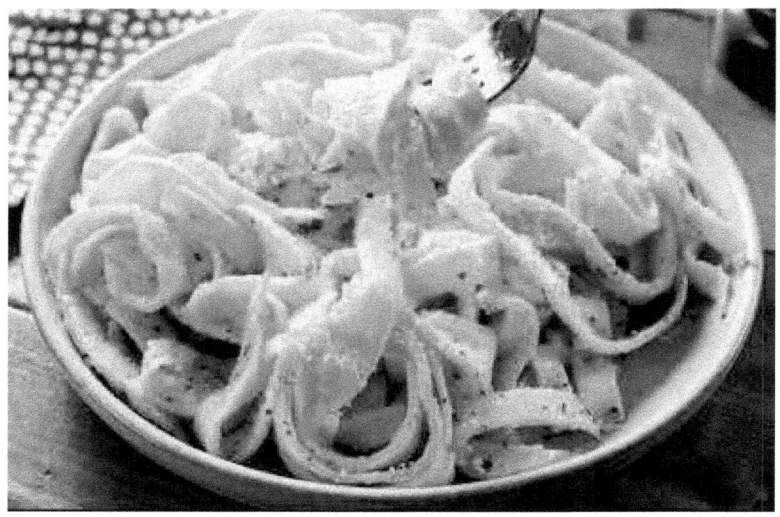

This recipe's literal magic, and will undoubtedly make the keto diet regimen easier than you can ever imagine. Cacio E Pepe is one of our perpetuity favorite pasta meals. This lightened up different varieties for making your pasta from scratch, and the good news is it's so much less complicated than it seems. All you need is an excellent nonstick pan.

Ingredients.

- 4 large eggs.
- Kosher salt.
- 2 tsp. Canola oil.
- 1 tbsp. Butter.
- 1/4 c. newly grated Parmesan for serving.
- Freshly ground black pepper.

Steps

- Break eggs right into a tool bowl period and add salt. Blend until smooth.
- In a nonstick skillet over medium-high heat 1 tsp oil. Add half the egg combination and twirl the frying pan to layer the bottom of the skillet with egg uniformly. Cook, continuously, until edges are formed, about 1 minute.
- Run a spatula along edges of egg to release, then use your hands to flip the omelet gently.
- Cook till egg is just set on the bottom, concerning 20 seconds.
- Slide omelet onto a cutting board and also allow cool slightly for 1 min. At the same time, repeat the process with remaining oil and eggs.
- Roll omelets up like a cigar and also cut right into 1/4- inch thick "noodles."
- Return skillet to medium-high and melt butter. While whisking, slowly gather 1/4 cup water until incorporated. Include Parmesan and pepper, and also stir till Parmesan melts into the sauce. Include noodles and also throw to coat.
- Season with even more pepper and also spray with more Parmesan before eating.

Zoodle Alfredo With Bacon.

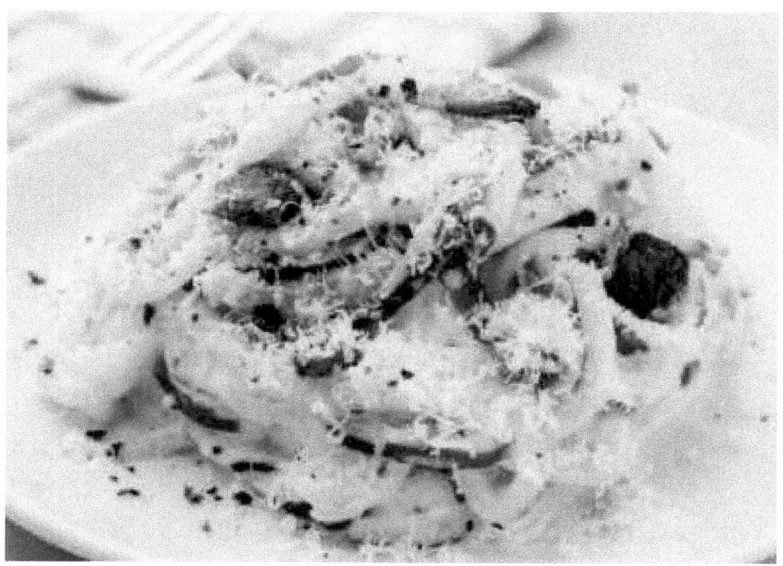

Ingredients.

- 1/2 lb. Bacon, sliced.
- 1 shallot, cut.
- 2 cloves garlic, diced.
- 1/4 c. gewürztraminer.
- 1 1/2 c. heavy cream.
- 1/2 c. grated Parmesan cheese, plus extra for garnish.
- 1 (16 oz.) container zucchini noodles.
- Kosher Salt.
- Newly ground black pepper.

Steps

- In a big frying pan over medium heat, cook bacon until crunchy, 8 mins. Drain on a paper towel-lined plate.
- Pour off all but 2 tbsps. Of bacon, then add shallots. Prepare up until soft, concerning 2 mins, then include the garlic and also chef until aromatic, regarding 30 secs. Add a glass of wine and also cook until lowered by half.
- Include whipping cream and also bring the mix to a boil. Reduce warm to reduced and stir in Parmesan. Prepare until the sauce has actually enlarged slightly, about 2 mins. Add zucchini noodles and also toss-up until completely coated in sauce.
- Get rid of it warmth and also stir the cooked bacon.

Tuscan Spaghetti Squash.

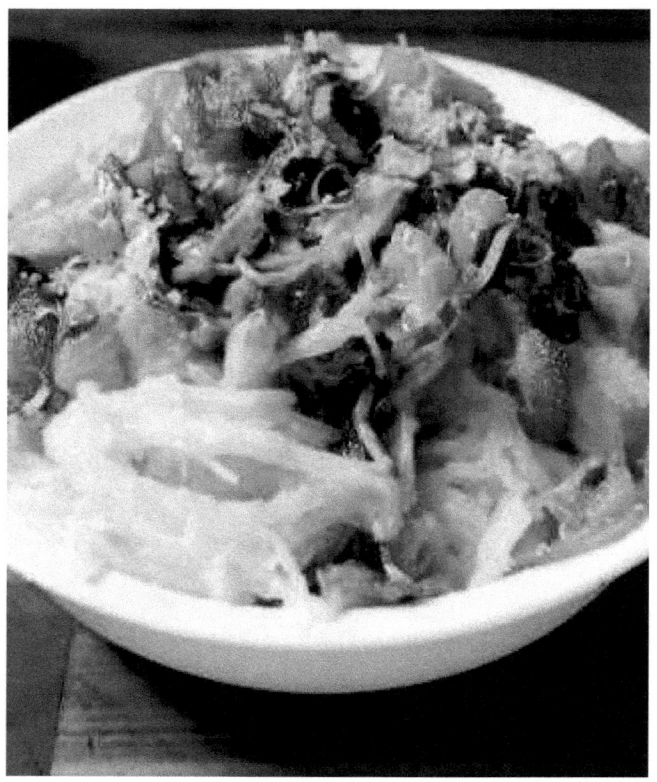

Ingredients

- 1 large spaghetti squash.
- 1 tablespoon. Extra-virgin olive oil.
- Kosher salt.
- Newly ground black pepper.
- 4 slices of bacon.
- 2 cloves garlic, minced.
- 1 1/2 cherry tomatoes, cut in half.
- 2 baby spinach.

- 1/2 whipping cream.
- 1/3 grated Parmesan.
- Basil, for garnish.

Steps.

- Preheat oven to 400 degrees F.
- Cut squash in half lengthwise. Scrub around with olive oil as well as a season with salt and pepper. Place the flesh side down on the baking sheet. Cook for 40-45 mins, until the pasta squash soft. Allow to cool until it is enough to deal with; after that, use two forks to rive pasta squash flesh into fine noodle- like strings.
- Meanwhile, cook bacon in a tool frying pan until crispy. Transfer to a paper towel-lined plate to drain.
- Pour off half the bacon fat and also add garlic, tomatoes as well as spinach to the frying pan—season with salt and pepper. Add whipping cream and Parmesan and let simmer up until somewhat thickened. Add pasta squash and toss-up until completely coated—Breakdown bacon over the squash as well as stir to combine.
- Garnish with basil.

CONCLUSION

One of the primary keys to any kind of successful diet regimen or way of living has continuously been the recipes that harmonize the principles of the diet regimen. I am sure there are several ways to accomplish ketosis, as well as to achieve that weight reduction objective. Nevertheless, you most definitely do not wish to get there by only having the same old meals over and over once more.

Selection is nitty-gritty below, which is essential in making sure the sustainability of the ketogenic diet. With the delicious and also scrumptious recipes found in this step by step keto cookbook, they will serve enhancements for any keto dieter at any phase of their ketogenic trip.

For the newbies that have gotten this recipe cookbook, it would be rather beneficial for you to take dish plan as a useful overview, but you must undoubtedly step out from that convenience area sooner or later as you progress along your keto adventure! This is what the several dishes are for so that you can pick and choose those that are most appealing to your taste.

This book and its components would have certainly been able to provide you detailed, actionable value for your progression towards nutritional ketosis. Much more notably, it is my hope that the book has additionally given you the self-confidence booster and has accumulated your commitment to remain on the diet regimen.

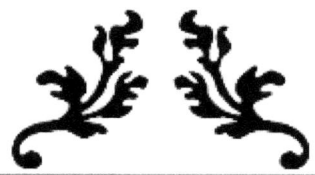

SOURDOUGH BREAD BAKING

Guide To Learn The Secrets Of Bread, How To Start Step By Step Sourdough, Quick And Easy Recipes

JULIA ROSS

PART ONE

THE PROCESS OF BAKING BREAD AND THE SOURDOUGH STARTER

Facts About Bread
Does the bread make you fat?

Thanks to many dietary trends in recent years, carbohydrates such as Rice, Potatoes, and Pasta have earned some bad press, and many of us are now skeptical of how much we eat these types of food. However, it is often more about what you spread, pour-over, or cook on these foods, which results in a high-calorie intake than the diet itself. For example, if you choose a wholemeal form that has more fiber than white bread, it will help you fuel up for longer, making you less likely to snack between meals. Take it a step further by preparing the loaf yourself, so you know what ingredients you're eating. You can either cook your bread in the oven or use a bread maker.

Why is Bread Moldy?

Molds are a form of fungi, and their spores are floating in the air all around us. Because the mold proliferates in dry, moist, and dark areas when it lands on bread, it can have the perfect environment to flourish on. The pattern can then replicate by sending more spores into the air, and in no time will your bread be filled with an unsightly grey / greenish growth.

So how can you avoid the moldy bread? Essentially, you need to do all you can to keep it dry and calm. Most people are trying to do this by putting it in the fridge. I notice that this helps to dry out too much of the bread. Also, you can freeze your food and unfreeze anytime to eat, and you want to consume it. Great for toasting but not as good for sandwiches as the bread can be left moist during defrosting. The other choice is to invest in a suitable bin of bread. It seems to me, having researched this, that a terracotta or grazed crock is a better choice than a wooden drawer. This is because those sly little spores will hole up in the warm wood and pop out when you place them in a nice fresh loaf.

Benefits Of Bread

Nothing may be compared to the aroma of freshly baked bread, and I prefer the taste of homemade loaf to that of a supermarket. That said, the ease of buying loaf means that many people still buy commercially baked bread from their convenience store and miss out on the advantages of a home-baked dough. I think it's fair to say that most people would prefer the taste and feel of the baked loaf. The crust is often better when the bread is baked in the oven.

Virtually infinite combinations of different flours and varying ratios of ingredients have resulted in various types of loaves of bread in shapes, sizes, colors, and textures.

As a simple food in the world, bread has become more critical than pure nutrition, becoming a staple in religious rituals, secular cultural life, and culture.

Below are some benefits of bread consumption:

Protein

Most people don't know bread is the third-largest protein contributor to our daily diet? Protein is essential to the growth, development, and repair of the body.

Fat

Bread naturally has low fat and is part of a healthy, balanced diet. It's what you're applying to your slice of bread, which needs to be monitored.

Carbohydrates

The bread is rich in complex carbohydrates. Carbohydrates are an essential part of our diet, supplying us with energy.

Vitamins B

The bread contains a variety of B vitamins, including thiamin (vitamin B1) and niacin (vitamin B3), which are essential for the release of energy from food.

Iron

Iron is a crucial element in wheat flour and is necessary for the production of red blood cells, which helps carry oxygen around the body and is vital for brain function.

Calcium

Calcium is well known for its role in the production of good teeth and healthy bones, and it is also essential for the proper functioning of the nerves, muscles, kidneys, and heart. Calcium is particularly vital in teenage and young adult years, as it is the period that our body builds up the maximum bone mass. Pat's Pan flour is enriched with calcium carbonate and contributes to the healthy development of young people and the maintenance of a healthy diet during their lifetime.

Types of bread

There are hundreds of different kinds of bread in the country. Note the subtle differences that may or may not be aimed at confusing the user.

White bread is manufactured from refined flour, i.e., grain from which the bran and germ have been separated so that it contains only the endosperm (the center of the grain). On the other side, wholemeal bread is made from the whole grain of wheat (endosperm, bran, and germ), i.e., from unrefined flour.

Brown bread is not the same thing as wholemeal bread. Also, brown bread is nothing more than white bread, to which a (usually caramel-based) coloring that has been applied to make it brown; up to 10% of bran can also be added.

Wholegrain bread is known to contain the whole grains, which have been included to increase the fiber content.

Granary bread it's made with a mixture of whole wheat and white flours, with cracked grains of malted barley and wheat.

Wheat germ bread is any type of bread to which a wheat germ has been added for flavoring.

Rye bread is bread made from rye instead of wheat. It possesses more fiber than most other breeds, darker color, and a better flavor.

Flatbreads are made from unleavened flour, water, and salted dough, although some are made with yeast. Flatbreads are particularly common in India.

Understanding Cereals
The World of Cereals
In their natural, unprocessed, wholegrain form, cereals are a rich source of vitamins, minerals, carbohydrates, fats, oils, and protein. In some developing nations, cereal in the form of rice, wheat, millet, or maize makes up a majority of daily sustenance. In developed countries, cereal intake is moderate and varied but still significant.

Cereals are among the earliest forms of benefiting foods, representing a victory in packaging, marketing, and diplomacy.

Unlike the majority of Europe, the UK has succumbed to the American cereal creation entirely. Approximately 100 years ago, natural grains, such as porridge or bread, were the staple breakfast seen around the world. Today, nevertheless, the Irish and British are the biggest consumers of puffed, flaked, sugared, salted, and extruded cereals on the planet!

Cornflakes (initially made by John Harvey Kellogg as a remedy for constipation) are made by reducing corn into smaller grits and steam cooking under pressure. The highly nutritious germ containing the vital fats is discarded as it goes rancid in time and interferes with the items shelf life. Flavorings, sugar, vitamins (to replace those removed) are added. They are after that rolled into flakes and toasted before being dried for packaging.

Frosted versions have sugar/ corn syrup and vitamins sprayed on the finished product. If you buy the economy variation of cornflakes, you are purchasing the fine dust left from the milling process, which is turned into pellets and shaped into flakes! These very same techniques and methods apply to all cereals in one way or another.

Cereal shapes are made from flours, which are mixed with water and heated up. Vitamins, having been damaged in the heating procedure, are added back into the flour mixture along with sugar salt and flavorings.

Many of the health benefits declared for breakfast cereals originate from added fortification rather than micronutrients from the raw ingredients, which are usually destroyed in the processing or removed ahead of time.

Flour is a form of powder made by grinding raw grains, nuts, roots, seeds, or beans. Cereal flour is the primary active ingredient of bread, which is an essential food for the majority of cultures. Wheat flour is one of the crucial components in the European, Oceanic, South American, North American, North Indian, Middle Eastern, and North African cultures. It is the defining component in their designs of bread and pastries.

Cereal flour consists either of the bran, germ, and endosperm together (wholegrain flour) or the endosperm alone (refined flour). The word "meal' is either differentiable from 'flour' about the somewhat coarser particle size (degree of comminution) or used as synonymous with flour; the word has used both ways. For instance, the word cornmeal often implies a grittier texture, whereas corn flour implies a fine powder, although there is no codified dividing line.

Types of Cereals

WHEAT

The term "cereals" is used for two things-- for "breakfast cereals" and as a synonym for "grains." Both will be looked at in this book.

Cereal emanates from "Ceres," which was the ancient Roman goddess of farming, is essentially lawn but cultivated and grown for the edible parts of its grain. They serve as a rich source of minerals, vitamins, carbohydrates, oils, fats, and protein if they are as whole gran (which is their natural type). If they are fine-tuned, they lose most of their useful parts and are left with carbohydrates.

Some of the world cereals include:

- Maize – (also referred to as corn) is a staple food of people in the Americas and Africa > It is also used as food for animals around the world.

- Rice – It grows in tropical and some temperate parts of the world. It is an essential food source in many locations of the world like South Asia, Latin America, and the far East. It has one of the highest worldwide production, alongside sugarcane and corn.

- Wheat - mainly grows in temperate areas, and it is a staple food there.

- Barley - Where corn can not grow, it is most likely that barley can. It is usually cultivated for malting and as food for animals.

- Sorghum – It is a staple food in Asia and Africa, specifically among the bad. It is also utilized as food for animals.

- Oats - when accessible worldwide as a winter season breakfast food and food for livestock, it is today used in cereals and is well-known for that.

- Rye - grown in a cold environment and used for cooking and as an active ingredient in alcohol.

Breakfast cereals can be classified into five categories:

- **Hot Cereals** - served and consumed hot; they can be wholesome and unsweetened sugary and processed. Unsweetened variation is healthier, and it can be enriched with much healthier versions like honey and fruit.
- **Whole-Grain Cereal**: It is healthier because it has many more vitamins, minerals, and other useful stuff for the human body. It can help lower cholesterol and sugar in the blood and avoid overindulging, to name a few things.
- **Bran Cereal** – It has much higher quantities of insolvable fiber. It helps food digestion and prevents constipation. It likewise provides filling of satiety, which lasts longer, getting rid of the requirement for food for a longer time.
- **Sugary Cereal--** cereal with high (sometimes expensive) sugar content, it is highly processed (which indicates not much of beneficial ingredients is in there), and has large quantities of preservatives and additives.

- **Organic Cereal**-- an inaccurate term, however, nevertheless utilized to describe cereals that don't use pesticides, artificial fertilizers, and no genetically customized ingredients. Their sweeteners are likewise natural (like honey for circumstances).
-

A few of the most popular breakfast cereals include:

- Frosted Flakes (by Kellogg's).

- Cap'n Crunch (by Quaker Oats).

- Lucky Charms (General Mills).

- Honey Nut Cheerios (General Mills).

- Cinnamon Toast Crunch (General Mills and Nestlé).

- Froot Loops (Kellogg's).

- Apple Jacks (Kellogg's).

- Cap'n Crunch's Crunch Berries (Quaker Oats).

- Rice Krispies (Kellogg's).

- Cocoa Puffs (General Mills).

- Raisin Bran (Kellogg's).

- Corn Pops (Kellogg's).

Ingredients For Bread Making

There is nothing more amazing than the scent of newly baked bread coming from the oven and wafting through space. There's no secret about bread baking, and it's one of the most useful things to do, even though the majority of individuals may believe that bread baking is a difficult task.

Of all, bread baking is a chemical process that involves the use of wheat gluten (flour), yeast for growing, a sweetener to feed the yeast, and warm water to supply a moist environment for the yeast and to tie the other components together. There are, therefore, just four essential ingredients to make a loaf of bread: flour, water, yeast, and sugar.

Flour

- Plain Flour

Plain flour is made by mixing well picked sturdy and soft wheat and is the finest fit for making bread and cakes.

- Whole Wheat Flour.

Bread made from whole wheat flour is typically little in size. A lot of wheat bread recipes blend entire wheat flour and bread flour to produce the best outcomes.

- Black Wheat Flour.

Black wheat flour also is called "raw flour," which is a high fiber flour that is very comparable to whole wheat flour. It must be utilized in conjunction with a high percentage of bread flour to accomplish a large size after growing.

- Oatmeal Flour and Corn Flour

Oatmeal is a product obtained by grinding the seeds of oats, preceded by the separation of the bran, which is rich in indigestible cellulose for the human organism. Oatmeal, although very rich in proteins, does not contain those that form gluten, which makes it, it is used alone, an ingredient not very suitable for the production of leavened foods, such as bread. Corn (or maize) represents one of the large agricultural productions of our country. Most are intended for zootechnical use (82%), while a small percentage is used for other applications (18%), including human nutrition. The beans still on the ear are consumed boiled or grilled, and those of some varieties "burst," giving rise to the crunchy popcorn.

Sweeteners.

Widely used in bread are sugar, honey, molasses, and malt powder, or merely enable the yeast to extract its nutrition from the sugar frequently found in the flour.

- Sugar.

Sugar is vital for adding flavor and color to the mix. (In my viewpoint, I do not believe sugar is needed.) as you can make sugar-free loaves, and I can't discriminate in taste or color. Sugar helps to feed the yeast to make better growing bread.

If you're using a bread maker, you might wish to search for components in your grocery store that say "excellent for bread makers." I seem to believe that those ingredients that come marketed for bread makers are of various quality than those used for regular baking.

Yeast.

Yeast breaks down and then produces co2, which expands the bread and softens the inner fiber. Yeast also depends on sugar and flour as a food source.

Yeast must likewise be kept at a cold temperature so that the fridge is the ideal place for storage.

Salt.

Salt is necessary to improve the taste of bread and the color of the crust. The presence of salt in the dough slows down the activity of the enzymes and, thanks to its ability to absorb water, the dough will be less sticky and more elastic. Salt acts positively on gluten, making the gluten mesh more resistant

Egg.

Eggs can enhance the consistency of your rice, include food, and make it bigger.

Grease, Butter, and Vegetable Oil.

Grease will soften the bread and prolong its service life. Before use, the butter should be melted or chopped into small pieces.

Baking Powder.

Baking Powder is generally utilized to make the bread increase quickly. Bubble or soften the consistency of the crust. Baking Soda The very same idea as above and the two can be used in combination with each other.

Liquid.

Water is an essential ingredient required in the process of making bread, so never leave it out of your dish. Liquid offers a growing medium for the yeast and serves as a binder to the other active ingredients. Fresh milk should be heated until it is utilized for making bread, as the enzymes in the milk inactivate the yeast and prevent the dough from increasing to its complete capability.

Essential Equipment

You're prepared to wade into the vast, fantastic world of bread making. Your cooking area is not entirely geared up?

Stress not, this section of the book to help you navigate the requirements so that you can focus your energy on accomplishing the ideal knead. We understand that baking your bread in the house can be intimidating enough without having to find out which tools are necessary, and which equipment provides the best value!

Many tools are used to make bread with excellent consistency and aroma. Some are useful and essential from the start; others can wait when you feel ready to use them. We've assembled a helpful list of breadmaking requirements to streamline your shopping, along with a couple of little luxuries that will prove well worth the investment over time, as your bread practice grows.

The most vital part is that each of these accessories can be utilized for a lot more than making bread! You'll enjoy discovering that they all can be found in useful in every aspect of cooking, both sweet and mouth-watering. Because actually, who has the area for tools that can't carry out a wide variety of functions?

Here are the required and essential tools I utilize to craft delicious gluten-free bread.

- Loaf Pan: Metal, non-stick, 9 inches by 5 inches.
- Rimmed Baking Sheet: Also called half-sheet pan metal pan with edges a minimum of 1 inch high.
- French Bread Pan: Metal pan with 3-or 4-inch-wide grooves. Might be perforated.

- Hamburger Bun Pan: Metal, non-stick, with 4-inch indentations for making buns and rolls. Six 4-inch ramekins are a suitable replacement.
- Instant-Read Digital Thermometer: This tool can help you ensure, for example, that you are warming water to 110 ° F(not 120 ° F, which will get rid of the yeast). It is also helpful for confirming the internal temperature of baked loaves to ensure they are baked.
- Parchment Paper: Baking paper or bakery release paper is cellulose-based paper. It's used in baking as a disposable non-stick surface. It should not be confused with wax paper or waxed paper.
- Mixing Bowls: Various sizes.
- Dry And Liquid Measuring Cups: Dry cups ought to have level edges and no put spouts. Liquid cups should be transparent and have a put spout.
  - Measuring Spoons: Standard **sizes** are 1/8 teaspoon, 1/4 teaspoon, 1/2 teaspoon, one teaspoon, and one tablespoon. Cheaper sets will omit the 1/8 teaspoon

Elective Tools

These are elective for baking tasty bread, but they can be handy for specific preparations.

- Stand Mixer: Should include whisk and paddle devices. A hand mixer is an acceptable replacement.
- Pizza Stone Or Steel: For cooking pizza and flatbreads when a heated area is more useful to produce a crisp crust.

- Springform Pan: A cake pan is an appropriate option.
- Muffin Tin: Can likewise be utilized for a hamburger bun pan for Dinner Rolls.
- Popover Pan: For Popovers.
- Brioche Pan: For Brioche. Helpful for inspecting your oven's proofing temperature level in addition to cooking temperature level-- many ovens run a little hot or cold.
- Oven Thermometer:
- Pastry Brush: For brushing the dough with oil or egg wash.
- Rolling Pin: Used for presenting croissant dough. Kitchen Area Scale: For weighing active ingredients.

Leavening

Leavening is applying gas to the flour, producing bubbles that make it swell. This makes it lighter and more comfortable to chew the bread. Once flour and water are combined to create a dough, the starch, whose quantity in the dough is large, absorb the water and form the electrostatic bonds with gluten, creating a homogenous mash. When the mixture is leavened (i.e., the gas is added), the dough ' raises.' Then, when it sets, the bubbles will remain trapped in the dough.

There are several ways in which the dough can be leavened. Nevertheless, most forms of bread are leavened using biological agents containing micro-organisms that emit carbon dioxide as part of their life cycle. They're either yeasts or sourdough starters.

Yeast is fermenting some of the carbohydrates in the flour. This causes carbon dioxide bubbles, which cause the dough to rise. A form of leaven requires proof, i.e., a quiet time to allow the yeast to replicate and eat carbohydrates. Bread leavened with yeast has a distinctive flavor. The sourdough starter is a paste of flour and water containing yeast and lactobacilli obtained from the previous batch of dough. It works in the same way as yeast, creating bubbles, but it takes a lot more time to prove it than yeast. Sourdough bread has a tangy, sour taste. It is used for rye-based bread, where the yeast is not useful in leavening the dough.

Chemical leavened are chemical mixtures that emit carbon dioxide or other gasses as they react to moisture and heat.

The most famous is baking powder, a mix of carbonate or bicarbonate (usually sodium bicarbonate), and one or more acid salts.

Baking powder works by adding carbon dioxide gas to the dough when it is warm, producing bubbles that extend the wet mixture. It is used instead of yeast for bread, where the flavors of fermentation would be undesirable or where the dough lacks the elastic structure needed to hold the gas bubbles for more than a few minutes.

Because carbon dioxide is released more quickly through an acid-base reaction than through fermentation, the bread made by chemical leaven is called quick bread. Examples of fast food include Irish soda bread, banana bread, pancakes, carrot cakes, and muffins.

The big question for diabetics, of course, is whether the rising method has any effect on the glycemic index (GI) of the bread. The intuitive answer is that the GI value needs to worsen because it adds moisture to the matrix. But according to researchers in New Zealand, the leaven agents used to make bread do not affect the GI of the bread.

Bread Making Process.

I believe it's valuable to examine the process steps beyond the recipe format to keep the recipes understandable and concise. It motivates a better understanding of the techniques to present them separately from the dish itself. Given that the strategies are the same for all of the recipes, as soon as you get it, you can work with the whole book confidently. I motivate you to take a seat and read through this chapter before you begin; it's difficult to absorb this info when you are in the middle of making a bread or pizza dough recipe for the very first time.

STEP 1: AUTOLYSE THE FLOUR AND WATER

Autolyze is my initial step in mixing bread and pizza dough. The flour and water are mixed and left to rest from 15 minutes to 24 hours without adding salt and yeast. I suggest an autolyze duration of 20 to 30 minutes for the dishes in this book. Don't add the salt during the autolyze, as it will hinder water absorption by the flour, and one of the goals of this step is to permit total hydration of the meal before mixing the final dough.

Measuring

The autolyze action takes about 5 minutes of hands-on time for determining the flour and water and mixing them by hand. Position your empty 12-quart dough tub on the scale, zero the size, then add the weight of flour specified in the recipe's Final Dough Mix column. (Remember, the meal should be at room temperature level.).

It's easy to include excessive water, so instead of measuring the quantity of water straight into the dough tub with the flour in it, I determine it into an empty container, then put the right weight of water into the tub with the flour.

The most convenient method to distribute water is to utilize two containers. Keeping your thermometer handy, put one box under the tap and change the hot and cold water mix till the water in the box is at the target temperature, for instance, 95 ° F(35 ° C). Put the empty box on your scale, and put in water from the first container until you reach the weight of water called for in the dish. Be exact with the weighing. Being off by as little as 20 or 30 grams can make a massive difference in the consistency of the dough.

Utilizing Your Kitchen Scale.

Put your empty container on the scale, press the scale's "zero" button (in some cases labeled "tare"), and after the scales zeroes out, thoroughly put in the component up until you reach the wanted weight. When you have numerous elements to contribute to the container, such as two or three various sorts of flour, just push the "no" button after each addition.

Add the Flour and Water.

Working directly in the 12-quart dough tub, mix the flour and water with one hand only up until integrated. Your hand will get sticky with dough. Don't stress; you need to get used to using your hand as an implement. Although dough bits are sticking to you (simply like they would attach to a dough hook), keep mixing up until the flour and water are incorporated. Any dough clumps need to be pinched through with your hand. After blending, utilize your free hand to squeegee the dough that's stayed with your working hand into the tub. Put a lid on the container and let the dough rest for 20 to 30 minutes. You will know the autolyze mixture is ready when there are no longer any loose bits of dry flour noticeable in the dough tub.

Working with Water Temperature.

The objective is for the final mixed dough to have a temperature level of about 78 ° F(26 ° C) this seems to be the perfect temperature level for both gas production and taste advancement. The dough doesn't require to remain at 78 ° F(26 ° C) throughout its improvement; it just needs to start there. I evaluated these dishes in my house cooking area, which is usually around 70 ° F(21 ° C).

You are utilizing water. 95°F (35°C), flour at space temperature, and a 20-minute autolyze duration, once the dough was blended, it was usually best at 78°F (26°C) during winter. In the summertime, I ratchet the water temperature to 90 ° F(32 ° C) to get the same outcome. There is a relationship between the heat of the ingredient and the environment and the rest time of autolysis before proceeding with the last mixture.

Although I recommend a 20-to 30-minute autolyze, you can extend it to 40 or even 60 minutes if that's easier for you. However, the autolyze mixture will cool off more, so your final mix temperature will be lower, and you may need to adjust your water temperature to compensate. Simply do not use water above 110°F (43°C). (As you might recall, temperatures much warmer than that can eliminate the yeast.) If you miss the target last mix temperature level of 78 ° F(26°C), review the temperature of water you used and the timing of the autolyze period, then adjust next time. Dishes from this book that utilize a preferment (a poolish or biga) will seldom have a last mix temperature level of 78 ° F(26 ° C), especially if your home is cold in the evening. This is since a significant percentage of the dough includes the advancement, which has developed overnight and will, for that reason, is at room temperature level-- whatever the overnight temperature level of your home is.

When Not To Autolyze.

In this book, the only dishes that don't have an autolyze step are those made with poolish or biga, where half or more of the recipe's total flour is in the advancement. These doughs acquire advantages similar to those produced in the autolyze due to the long, overnight development of the improvement, which includes only a bit of yeast and no salt. Autolyzing dough made with poolish is also impractical. For this book's recipes that include a poolish, the extra active ingredients for the last dough mix contain only 250 grams of water, however, another 500 grams of flour, which would result in dough clumps that are impossible to exercise manually.

When To Hydrate The Yeast

Granular dried yeast takes longer to liquify in stiffer doughs (in my world, that would be hydration of 70 percent or less). Store-bought instant yeast is developed to work without being dissolved initially. However, that's based on the assumption that the dough will be mixed by a device, which integrates the active ingredients far more strongly than hand mixing does. We do not hydrate, or evidence, instant yeast at my bakery, however, that's because we typically utilize fresh yeast in our stiff doughs.

The very first time I hand combined an overnight biga (at 68 percent hydration) with instant yeast while testing a dish in this book, I was amazed by the lack of gassiness and rise in the biga the next early morning. Even with hand mixing, the high hydration ensures that the yeast granules dissolve totally and end up being active early in the dough's evolution. The exceptions are for biga (at 68 percent hydration) and pizza doughs (at 70 percent hydration).

STEP 2: MIX THE DOUGH

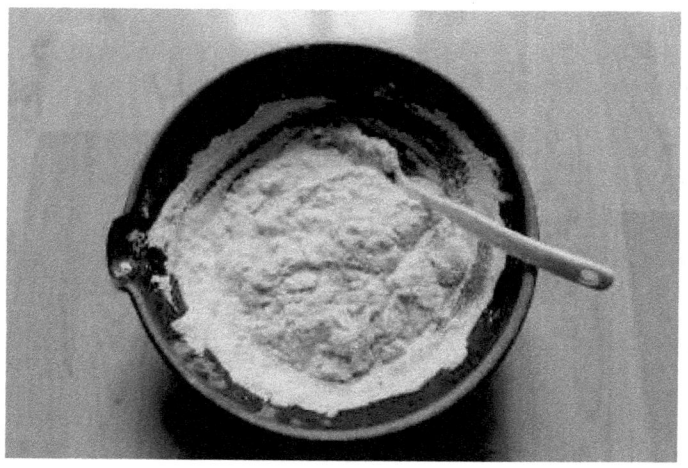

Hand mixing the final dough ought to take about 5 minutes. I prefer to mix it by hand in the dough tub, instead of kneading it on the counter or utilizing a mixer. It's easier, quicker, and involves less clean-up, and it's completely valid. The dough remains in the very same tub from the autolyze action till it is divided and formed into loaves about 5 or 6 hours later, depending on the dish. No hassle, no muss!

Add the Salt and Yeast

To mix the dough, do not put salt and yeast together because the salt counteracts the action of the yeast.

Establish a container of warm water next to your dough station. Hold the dough tub by the rim with your weaker hand and wet your more powerful hand in the warm water. Begin to blend by reaching underneath the dough and getting about one-quarter of the mixture. Stretch this area of dough, then fold it over the leading to the other side of the mix.

When folding segments of dough, extend them out to the point of resistance, then fold them back throughout the whole length of the dough mass. Working your way around the mixture, repeat with the staying quarters of the dough, reaching underneath each time.

Use the Pincer Method

Once all of the dough has been folded over itself, continue blending utilizing the pincer approach. Using a pincerlike grip with your thumb and forefinger, capture huge portions of dough and then tighten your grip to cut through the dough. Do this consistently, working through the whole mass of dough. With your other hand, turn the tub while you're blending to provide your active side with an excellent angle of attack.

Dip your blending hand back into the container of warm water three or four times throughout this procedure to rewet it and prevent the dough from staying with you. The dough will be sticky and tough to work if you don't. It is normal to feel the granularity of the salt and yeast as you blend; utilizing a wet hand for mixing will assist the salt and yeast dissolve.

Cut through the dough five or six times with the pincer approach, then fold it over itself a few times, then once again cut through it five or six times and fold over itself a few more times. Repeat this procedure, rotating between cutting and folding, until you see and feel that all of the active ingredients are completely integrated, and the dough has some tension in it. For me, this takes 2 or 3 minutes. It might take 5 or 6 minutes when you're brand-new at this. Let the dough rest for a couple of minutes, then fold for another 30 seconds or till the mixture tightens up. That's it for blending!

The objective of this step is to include all of the components thoroughly. It efficiently incorporates the ingredients and disperses the salt and yeast throughout the mix. At the end of the mix, determine the temperature level of the dough with a probe thermometer. In the majority of the recipes in this book, the target temperature level is 77 ° F to 78 ° F(25 ° C to 26 ° C). Write down the last mix temperature and time. If the dough temperature is well below 77 ° F(25 ° C), it will take longer to increase, in which case you'll need to follow the recipe guidelines relating to just how much the dough should broaden, rather than the suggested time. You can compensate by placing the dough tub in a warm area for the increase 75 ° F to 80 ° F(24 ° C to 27 ° C) ought to work. Use warmer or colder water next time if your mix temperature was listed below or well above 78 ° F (26 ° C).

Letting the Dough Rise Cover the tub and let the dough increase. The quantity of time this takes depends on lots of elements, especially the final mix and the ambient temperature. Relate to the visual hints in the recipe as your target, keeping in mind that your dough will have a little bit more volume in warmer months and a little less volume in colder months.

STEP 3: FOLD THE DOUGH
Folding the dough helps develop the gluten that provides the mixture its strength and adds to significant volume in

the last loaf. Think about the three-dimensional web of gluten as the frame of the bread "house." For the first dish, the Saturday White Bread, simply two folds are required. The majority of the other bread doughs have higher hydration, and much of these slack doughs take advantage of 3 or 4 folds to provide the strength they require. Each fold takes about 1 minute. You'll have the ability to acknowledge when to apply the next fold based on how unwinded the dough has become: it goes from being a ball with a structure to lying flattened out in the tub. With each fold, it companies up a bit. I try to operate in all the folds during the first hour or more of the increase.

The action here is simply like the folding throughout blending in step 2, but after folding, you'll invert the dough to help it hold its tension. To fold the dough, dip your active hand in the container of warm water to wet it, so the dough does not stick to you. With your moistened hand, reach beneath the mixture and pull about one-quarter of it out and approximately extend it up until you feel resistance, then fold it over the leading to the opposite of the dough. Repeat four or five times, working around the mixture until the mixture has tightened up into a ball. Get the entire ball and invert it so the seam side, where all of the folds have come together, deals with down. This assists the folds to hold their position. The top needs to be smooth.

When the dough relaxes a bit and flattens in the bottom of the tub, repeat the process for the second fold. After each fold, the dough develops more structure or strength than it had in the past and will, therefore, take longer to unwind totally. You can do any subsequent folds called for in the recipe an hour or two later, or you can give the dough all of its folds in the very first hour after blending, whatever is hassle-free for you. Just do not fold the dough during the last hour of bulk fermentation.

STEP 4: DIVIDE THE DOUGH

When the dough has doubled or tripled (whichever is defined in the dish), it's time to divide it. When bulk fermentation is complete, one of the factors clear Cambro tubs are so useful for bread making is that they enable you to identify rapidly. For instance, if a dough needs to triple in size throughout bulk fermentation and it begins at a little bit more than 1 quart, it should come up to nearly the 4-quart line once tripled. This action will take simply a couple of minutes when you've done it a couple of times. In the beginning, it may take a little bit longer.

Gently flour a work surface area; you'll need a location about 2 feet wide. Working beside the floured site, flour your hands and gently loosen up the dough around the border of the tub, making sure not to let the gluten strands tear. (At this point, the gluten is more fragile than it was when the dough was first mixed.) Reach to the bottom of the tub and gently loosen the bottom of the dough from the container. It's practical to toss some flour along the edges to work beneath the dough and help alleviate its release. Then turn the box on its side and utilize your hands to assist gently relieve the mixture out onto the work surface area. Sprinkle flour across the middle of the top of the dough, where you'll suffice, then divide it into two equal-size pieces with a dough knife, plastic dough scraper, or cooking area knife.

STEP 5: SHAPE THE LOAVES

The goal of shaping the dough into loaves is to protect and keep the gas formed during the leavening inside.

Be conscious that when your dough pieces are resting on the floured work surface, the underside of the dough will become beyond the loaf; this will help you comprehend the shaping process. The bottom of each piece of dough is resting on some flour, so it's not going to be as sticky there. Keeping your hands in contact with that part of the mixture is the most important guidance I can provide; otherwise, the dough will stay with your hands.

Begin by brushing any loose flour off the top of the dough with your hand. Then, utilizing the same method as in the folding action, stretch and fold one-quarter of the mixture at a time up and over the leading to form around, carefully pulling each sector out up until you get to its maximum stretch, then folding it over the prominent to the opposite side. Repeat, working your way around the dough and forming it into a ball, till the interior is enclosed and you have around with a little stress in it. Flip it over, so the seam is on the work surface in a location cleared of flour at this point, you want the friction, or grip, of a clean surface area.

Cup your hands around the back of the dough ball as you face it. Pull the entire dough ball 6 or 8 inches towards you on the dry, not covered in flour surface, leading with your pinky fingers and using sufficient pressure, so the dough ball grips your work surface and doesn't just slide throughout it. As you pull, this will tighten up the ball and add tension to it. You can feel it. It feels good.

Give the loaf a quarter turn and repeat this tightening action. Continue in this method till you've gone all the way around the dough ball two or three times. The loaf does not require to be incredibly tight, but you do not want it to be loose, either. I am trying to find enough tension so that the loaf holds its shape and its gases. If the shaped loaves are too soft, without adequate stress, there's a less physical structure to hold on to the gases. Some gas will get away, resulting in bread that's smaller and a bit much heavier than the ideal.

Also, mold the second piece of dough and place both loaves with the seam downwards in a suitable container: these bread baskets are dusted with flour or covered with fabric that can be scattered. You need to use sufficient flour so that the proofed loaf can be removed without sticking, but not a lot that you wind up with a lot of excess powder on the loaf. Lightly flour the top of the shaped loaves and cover with a kitchen towel or put the proofing baskets in nonperforated plastic bags.

STEP 6: PROOF THE SHAPED LOAVES
In the baking industry, the term proofing is commonly used to describe the final rise, after the loaf is shaped. (It is likewise utilized to refer to hydrating yeast before the dough mix;.) To attain the full capacity of your loaves, you require to evidence them entirely. The loaves need to reach their physical limit for hanging on to their gases before the gluten network starts to break down as the proteins degrade in time. Bake too quickly, and you lose the last smidgen of taste and volume development the bread can, and the loaves will be too tight and will bloom unevenly.

Bake too late (overproof), and the loaves will deflate, losing and collapsing volume.

Forming the loaves.

Very first row: Stretching a sector of dough and folding it over itself.

2ND row: Stretching the 2ND section of dough and folding it over itself.

3rd row: Folding the final segment of dough over itself.

Fourth row: Cupping hands around the back of the dough ball and pulling it throughout the not covered in flour work surface area; a completed dough ball.

One mark of a seasoned baker is the ability to bake the bread at that ideal point of the proof each time, and it stays a regular topic of conversation at my bakeshop. It's not simple for bread, however, for croissants and brioche, too. We learn by doing, and often the most excellent method to discover is to be ready to have a loaf that's a bit over- proofed. This will help you comprehend what the limitations are.

The Finger-Dent Test

To do the test, poke the increasing loaf with a floured finger, making an imprint about 1/2 inch deep. The loaf needs more proofing time if it springs back instantly. The loaf is proofed and prepared to bake if the indentation springs back gradually and incompletely. The loaf is over-proofed if the imprint doesn't spring back at all. You've waited too long, and the loaf may collapse a bit when you eliminate it from its basket or put it into the Dutch oven for baking. You can extend that window by proofing these bread overnight in the refrigerator. The cold dough will develop more slowly, offering you a window of proofing approximately a couple of hours.

STEP 7: PREHEAT THE OVEN AND DUTCH OVEN

Position a rack in the middle of the oven. If you bake too close to the bottom of the oven, you risk scorching the bottom of the loaves. Put your 4-quart Dutch oven inside with the lid on. There is no requirement to place the Dutch oven on a pizza stone; the cast-iron mass serves a similar purpose—Preheat the oven to 475 ° F(245 ° C) for a minimum of 45 minutes. The goal is for the Dutch oven to be filled with oven heat before you place the loaf inside.

It's essential to understand your oven. The majority of house ovens run hotter or colder than the temperature level you set them to. Mine runs about 25 ° F cooler, so when I set it to 500 °F. I get 475 ° F. The temperatures given up the dish are, of course, the actual temperature level the bread needs to be baked at, so I advise that you use an oven thermometer. They just cost a few dollars, and utilizing one will ensure you that you're cooking at the correct temperature, permitting you to follow the recommended baking times with self-confidence.

If you have 2 Dutch ovens and can fit both of them in the oven at the same time, preheat both of them. Each recipe offers particular directions on how to store the second loaf while the first one bakes if you only have one Dutch oven. Generally speaking, if your loaves proof at room temperature level, you should put the 2Nd loaf in the refrigerator someplace around 15 to 20 minutes before baking the very first loaf. If your loaves proof in the fridge overnight, keep the 2ND loaf in the refrigerator while the very first loaf is baking. When the very first loaf comes out of the oven, reheat the Dutch oven for about 5 minutes before baking the 2ND loaf.

STEP 8: BAKE-- VERY CAREFULLY

All of the bread in this book bake in covered preheated Dutch ovens for 30 minutes at 475 ° F(245° C), then the lid is removed while the bread completes baking, generally 15 to 20 minutes longer. Each dish specifies baking times. When dealing with Dutch ovens, I heartily suggest using oven mitts instead of kitchen towels or hot pad. Oven mitts go partway up your forearms, providing higher protection from the high heat of the Dutch oven and its cover. I act with higher self-confidence when wearing oven mitts and motivate you to use them. As soon as a Dutch oven runs out the stove, I discover it useful to put the gloves on the hot lid manage so I won't absentmindedly pick it up without first placing a glove back on. Take every preventative measure.

To move the dough from the proofing basket to the Dutch oven, first thoroughly invert the proofed loaf from its basket onto a floured countertop, bearing in mind that the top of the baked loaf will be the side that was facing down while it was rising. If the dough stays with the edges of the proofing basket, use one hand to delicately launch the mixture and make a mental note that you need to dust the basket with a bit more flour the next time. Preferably, the weight of the dough should cause it to reduce onto the countertop with no support. New wicker baskets need a little more flour than seasoned baskets, and they do not require to be cleaned up between usages.

Since the loaves are baked with the seam side up (the side opposite the smooth top of the shaped loaf in the proofing basket), and after a total proof, cracks will naturally open on the top of the loaf as it broadens in the oven.

Next, exceptionally carefully place the loaf in the hot Dutch oven. It's already resting on the counter best side up, so just carefully drop it into the Dutch oven without flipping it over. Utilize the sides of your bare hands to get the loaf and location it in the pot. Don't choose it up with your fingertips; it's fragile at this stage, and it's finest to spread out the pressure needed to pick it up across the dough. Use mitts to put the cover on the Dutch oven and place it in the preheated oven.

When you eliminate the lid after 30 minutes of baking, the loaf will be increased entirely, and you should see several attractive splits in the top where the dough expanded. The crust needs to have a light brown color. Use the time in the recipe as a guideline for how long to bake the loaf exposed, but be sure to examine about 5 minutes before the time has elapsed, so you're in tune with the loaf's development. Bake until dark brown all around the loaf. I like to bake until there are areas of extremely dark brown for the complete flavors those bits of crust have. At least as soon as, you should try baking a loaf just shy of the point of burning it, I'm wowed by the way these dark loaves taste and look. When the bread is baked, eliminate the Dutch oven from your kitchen area oven and tilt it to turn the loaf out. Let it cool on a rack or set on its side so air can distribute around it. Let the loaf rest for a minimum of 20 minutes before slicing. The within the loaf continues to bake after it's gotten rid of from the oven, and it needs that time to finish. Take pleasure in the crackling sound of the cooling bread.

Storing Baked Bread

I overcame my hostility to saving bread in plastic bags many years back, after trying all the options and understanding absolutely nothing else keeps the bread also. The crust will soften, but the bread will not dry. The straight dough bread will stay for two or three days. The bread made with preferments will hold a day longer than that, and the leavened bread from this book will continue for five to six days if you do not consume it all before then!.

Tips

- ✓ Apply folds to the dough to give it the wet strength mixtures require to hold their form.
- ✓ Push the fermentation to just shy of its limits to g the very best tastes.
- ✓ Bake the bread until it's a deep, dark brown.
- ✓ Keep a log of dough temperatures, fermentation times, and other information to assist you in fine-tuning your procedure.
- ✓ Retard leaving loaves after forming for at lest twelve hours, or use a long, overnight bulk dough fermentation.

Tips For Bread Making

Bread involves baking a mixture of flour, water, salt, yeast, and other active ingredients. The necessary procedure includes the blending of elements till the flour is converted into a stiff dough or paste, followed by baking the dough into a loaf.

The objectives of the breadmaking processes are to produce a dough that will increase quickly and have properties required to make great bread for the consumer.

To make excellent bread, dough made by any procedure needs to be extensible enough for it to unwind and to expand while it is increasing. When pulled, a good mixture is extendable if it stretched. It also needs to be elastic, that is, have the strength to hold the gases produced while rising and steady adequate to hold its shape and cell structure.

When blended with water, two proteins present in flour (gliadin and glutenin) form gluten. It is gluten that offers dough these unique residential or commercial properties. Gluten is necessary for bread making and affects the blending, kneading, and baking of residential or commercial properties of the mixture. When you first begin to make bread, finding out to blend the ingredients is crucial.

You can begin by putting a particular amount of warm liquid in a big blending bowl along with the sweetener and the amount of yeast. Generally enough, in a batch of dough that requires six cups of flour, 1 tbsp, or a single package of yeast. Offer the yeast to prove it for about 5-10 minutes. You're going to understand if the yeast is alive if it begins to grow and bubble. Discard it and purchase some new yeast if the yeast does not reveal any signs of presence. It's time to start applying the flour. The flour should be included in little increments and thoroughly mixed before the next addition. Typically, 1 cup of liquid will be enough to soak up about 6 cups of flour.

Something you should remember when making bread is that not all flours are the same and that the weather affects the absorption rate of flour. If there is a lot of moisture in the air, more flour will be required, and if it is scorched, less flour will be needed.

Once the dough has formed (which is not sticky but is soft enough to knead), it is time to put it on a floured surface and begin kneading it. You should use the heels of your hands (the firmest part above the wrist) for kneading the dough. Start from the top, lower your heels, and fold your fingers back. Simply knead it with your fingertips. Of all, there's not sufficient strength in your hands to knead the dough correctly, and second of all, when you begin kneading the dough, it's going to be weak and exuding through your fingers, making it an untidy and challenging job. As you press, add flour as required to keep the dough from sticking. The kneading process will take about 10 minutes.

When the dough is adequately kneaded, it will be smooth and elastic. This is when you press it, it will immediately go back to its initial position.

When you are sure that the dough is entirely kneaded, put it in a large greased bowl and cover with plastic wrap or a tidy towel. In warm days, the mixture will increase very rapidly, and in cold days it will take longer.

Once the dough has risen, beat it down and knead for about a minute. Enable to rest for about 5 minutes and after that shape a loaf or two if it is a large amount of dough. Typically speaking, 6 cups of flour will make a massive loaf of bread or two smaller ones. The bread can be put in greased loaf pans that have actually been sprayed with cornmeal or can be easily prepared on a flat baking sheet. In any case, ensure the containers are greased or sprayed with a vegetable spray. Cornmeal will function as a user interface that permits the bread to be quickly released from the pan. It also includes a texture of interest to the bread.

Permit the rounded loaf (covered with cling wrap or a clean towel) to grow in a warm place until it is doubled in size. Bake in a 375-degree oven for 25-45 minutes, depending upon the components and the size of the loaf. It ought to sound hollow when it's done if you tap the bottom of the baked loaf. You can likewise utilize an instant reading thermometer to inspect the inside of the bread. It's expected to reach 200 F. When it's done cooking. When the bread is done, remove it from the oven and let it cool. Turn the pan over (loaf pan) and position the bread on a cooling rack to complete the cooling procedure when it's cool enough to handle. If you bake the bread on a sheet of food, you can remove it with a big spatula.

Slicing hot bread is the most convenient way to do it with a hot knife. Your knife blade can be warmed by running it under a warm water tap. You should, nevertheless, allow your bread to cool off for a long time before slicing it like hot bread when sliced, which might tend to be gum. Cooling permits excess wetness to leave.

Guidelines You Need To Know Before Starting A
newly baked bread is as delicious as it is soothing, Baking
bread in the house goes beyond stretching resources and
preventing a trip to the grocery store, it's a method of doing
something positive for the family while you are home.

Kneading dough is likewise an excellent type of tension
relief, something a lot of people might discover comfort in
right now. As delicious as sourdough bread can be, just a
single mistake can be a frustrating waste of ingredients and
time.

- **How to knead perfectly?**

While some recipes are for no-knead bread, kneading
typically plays a considerable role in getting the texture in
the right way. When you knead the dough, work on a lightly
floured surface, fold the extreme side of the dough towards
you and, using you're the heels of your hand, press the
dough down, stretching it back. Turn the dough a quarter
and repeat."

After a few minutes, the mixture should be smooth and easy
compared to the initial sticky and floppy texture. To know if
your dough was kneaded properly, take a small portion, and
stretch it between your fingers, it should be able to slim
down without crumbling. If the mixture breaks down
extremely fast, just continue kneading.

- **Do not strain the dough**

When you are mixing your dough with your hand, it's
improbable that one may strain it. If, when you are
kneading the dough, it seems to withstand being extended

and exceptionally quickly bounces back, or you're having difficulty folding the dough onto itself, you're most likely verging on overworking the dough. Simply stop kneading, and your bread must still turn out merely beautiful.

- **Sticky dough is normal**

You might be afraid of how sticky it appears when you begin working with freshly combined dough. "Don't worry, and withstand the desire to add more flour to your mixture. The more flour you include, the heavier and tighter the inner of the bread will be. The moment you continue kneading your dough, the gluten strength will increase, and the dough will start to stay together more, and adhere to your hands and countertop less. When you notice it is still sticky and almost impossible to work with, put some oil on your hands. Don't add oil to the dough, only your fingers.

- **Proofing is powerful**

Proofing dough (allowing it to increase and rest) might look like an action people can skip when trying to save time; however, it's genuinely, actually important.

When making your dough, it should continuously feel energetic and alive with air and bubbles in it. It shouldn't have a rough and collapse texture, rather, it ought to be springy and supple,

Beginning bakers must follow whatever recipe they're utilizing as carefully as possible and, as they get comfier, can make changes on proofing time based on their preferred result.

- **Experimenting flavor**

As soon as you've nailed a fundamental bread dish, keep going. Raid your spice rack for spices blends to contribute to the dough. Or chop freshly chosen herbs and add them in. Try grating a lovely delicate cheese to add in, or chunk up a good cheddar and add newly chopped jalapeño peppers. When including tastes, the sky is the limit, so do not hesitate to get innovative.

- **Be patient**

Keep in mind that making bread is a procedure, so simply relax and take your time with it.

The Starter Sourdough Basics

Bakers have used wild fermentation for many centuries to leaven their bread. The very same procedure is at work when grapes are used to make wine. Vines are usually covered with the yeast considered suitable for making wine.

Flour and water are added, then give it some time, and you will end up with a sourdough starter that you can use to make the desired sourdough bread. Some bakers make a fresh sourdough starter or "levain" on a regular basis.

Microbiologically, once a starter is steady as well as maintained healthy, it does not get any much better with age. A little love with the tale of the family starter granny continued to live on the wagon train is perfectly fine. As long as the starter jobs generate great delicious bread as well as is healthy and balanced, it doesn't matter a lot.

Tips For Making And Caring For Your Sourdough Starter

A fascinating process is set in motion when you add water to some flour. The micro-organisms that survive the grain, which has been ground into flour, start to absorb the starches as well as sugars in the flour, generating gas as well as enzymatic activity.

This process is called fermentation. Fermentation renders flour a lot more digestible by damaging down Phytates existing in the grain and predigesting the gluten and also starch. During fermentation, hairs of gluten (called Glutenin and Gliadin), living in some grains, particularly in wheat, bond together, developing a sticky internet which traps gas bubbles and triggers dough to increase.

If you can't get a sourdough starter from someone, you can make your own. Making your sourdough starter is effortless and enjoyable; it merely takes a few ingredients as well as time (concerning two weeks).

Requirements For Making Sourdough Starter

• **Container**

For the container which you will use to maintain your sourdough starter, use a food quality plastic container (a huge yogurt container or plastic ware will do great), a crockpot or a bowl with a cover which can hold about 32-48 fluid ounces (around 2 quarts or 2 liters), something that will hold about 4 - 8 mugs. Do not utilize reactive steel execute to stir your starter with. You can use a glass container, yet there is a threat of getting items of glass in your sourdough starter if you accidentally hit the edge with something.

• **Flour**

The micro-organisms essential to get your starter fermenting are abundant in fresh flour, particularly rye and wholegrain flour. Bleached/bromated flour is not specifically valuable for making a starter; the chemicals can interfere with the procedure. Make a mixture of (50/50) white flour and some whole grain flour as well as store it in a container to feed your starter with.

- **Water**

Use distilled water. Attempt to use water that does not include chlorine or various other chemicals in it, ideally. The micro-organisms which make up the starter are delicate to chemicals. If you only have accessibility to tap water, set the faucet water out in a container overnight to allow the chlorine to escape. Gently cover the box with a towel to stay out dirt. You can use filtered water to make a starter. If you have to use water, attempt to obtain water that has not been distilled, the minerals in the water help maintain the starter healthily and balance.

- **Juice**

Juice can be made use of in a mixture of half juice as well as half water for the first four days to start your brand-new sourdough starter. Pineapple, orange or other types of juice include a level of acidity to the starter, and also aid motivates the proper micro-organisms to thrive.

- **Salt**

Since it can be used in small quantities to regulate over fermenting, Salt is pointed out right here. In warmer climates and also with some kinds of flour, a sourdough starter can have trouble fermenting too quickly. Salt helps control fermentation by preventing the chemical action (particularly Protease). If you can, Use sea salt or salt that has no chemical additives. There are many fantastic sea salts available on the marketplace currently. A good salt adds not only flavor but minerals to your baking products.

The Process Involved

When you blend flour and also water, numerous things happen. The flour ends up being moisturized, and the gluten hairs start to bond, microbes already present in the flour multiply, and even enzymes begin to damage down starches into sugars to feed the micro-organisms. The microbes are generally yeasts and bacteria. There can be numerous kinds of organisms present in the flour, yet the one you want to urge is the micro-organisms that thrive in acidic conditions (lactic add bacteria). During the initial four days after you make the flour and also water mix, the organisms defend prominence. After four days, the starter will naturally end up being a lot more acidic, as well as the correct micro-organisms develop themselves in their new residence. That is why throughout the first four days, when the microbes are combating for dominance, the starter can smell awful, like dirty socks.

Now, many bakers will throw the starter because they assume it spoiled. But it's just a phase on the trip. By day five or six, the starter begins to smell more yeasty as well as fruity as you expect it to. Don't offer up, keep feeding your starter as well as be a person. This is also the reason that using half water/half juice can help jumpstart the process. It helps the proper microbes establish themselves quicker.

Often during the procedure, you may observe that your sourdough starter scents like acetone or sharp. If that happens, it suggests you are not feeding it sufficient as well as you either need to feed the starter more food throughout feeding time, feed it a lot more usually, or both.

How to Create Sourdough Starter

Sourdough starter is made from flour and water. It does not end there; it consists of living yeast and bacteria making it to life as well as growing as you save it for lengthy periods.

As long as you keep it well fed, you will certainly have all the bread that you will need. As the yeast multiplies, it leavens your bread. To make the sourdough bread, you blend the starter with flour and make a dough.

To develop your starter, comply with these actions:

- Find a container where you can store your starter. Sourdough bakers recommend using a wide-mouthed glass jar. Utilizing a Tupperware of Rubbermaid container is also excellent. If you seem like reusing, make use of a wide-mouthed mayonnaise or pickle container. Since some of its components respond to the starter, be wary with making use of metal containers. It coincides with the utensils you utilize when mixing your starter, stay clear of metal ones.

You will require a mug of cozy water, a cup of flour, as well as a little bit of yeast (optional). Utilizing yeast can give an increase to your starter; however, your sourdough starter would certainly still be great without it.

- To allow the yeast currently existing in the flour to increase, keep the starter in a cozy place. To feed it, throw half the starter away and include a half mug of flour as well as a half mug of water to the half of the starter that is left. Feed your starter every day.

- Keep your starter in the fridge covered with a cover. See to it that it is not entirely airtight

Distinctions Between Sourdough and also Brewer's yeast

Yeast types are relatively well adjusted to their natural food resources. You would certainly have to feed it with the natural substrate for the yeast you're making use of, as well as when it comes to brewer's yeast, that's most likely malt of some type as well as you'll wind up with beer rather than a starter.

If you fed it flour (as we carry out in traditional sourdough), all that you would accomplish is this: over time, the all-natural wild yeast currently existing in your flour will certainly out-compete the maker's yeast. Also, you'll wind up with a traditional sourdough, not a "brewer's yeast" society. This is why it does not even help to include the baker's yeast to "leap begin" a starter. It will take longer for the wild yeasts in the flour to take hold and also establish your sourdough.

You probably can't make such radical "developer" cultures to bake with. There is, however, some variant based upon area and sort of flour. The starter made from rye flour expanded in Germany will likely have some different features than a wheat starter from San Francisco.

Having Enough Starter for Your Formula

If the formula calls for 100 grams of starter, then add 50 grams of flour as well as 50 grams of water to your starter the night before you prepare to utilize it. If you need a lot of starter for a massive batch of bread, don't put out any of the starters, simply feed the sourdough starter lots extra food and maintain it in a cozy or area temperature area.

Testing Your Starter's Capability

Years ago I established an experiment where I took every one of the starters I was maintaining at the time, and I evaluated them for the length of time it took them to double and also then the period until they came to a head (the most significant degree at which they fall back). I fed the starters as well as after that gauged the very same amount right into each jar as well as noted the level where the starter had risen each hr. It was interesting because the beginners had different capabilities or proofing times.

The standard or typical starter has excellent raising power for regarding 6 hours, starters with shorter abilities need to be made use of for quick bread and also one-day loaves. I have a starter that will undoubtedly come to a head in regarding ten hours, and that is a terrific starter for the extremely lengthy fermented doughs that I like to function with.

Do not be shocked if your starter falls back when it peaks,
„ yet then rallies as well as elevates up a tiny quantity once again. When you understand your starter's peak time, you can readjust your bulk ferment to take advantage of your beginner's capability. If your starter ferments as well rapid

as well as you desire to reduce it down, include a pinch of salt.

STARTER VARIATIONS

If you would like to have whole wheat or a rye starter or any kind of various other various types of starter, proceed to feed your starter every day, yet feed it with your favored flour instead of white flour. A well-established starter could reduce down if you alter its diet plan unexpectedly.

You will need to feed your starter every day to keep it healthy and balanced. You can refrigerate your new starter for short durations of time when it isn't being made use of, now that it is mature. When they want to bake, they will certainly take out their starter, feed it and keep it at space temperature until it is energetic once again, then utilize it for cooking with, feed it once more and also keep it in their refrigerator until they want to use it once again.

KEEP IN MIND: The over procedure is a natural means to begin your starter. Some bakers make use of pineapple juice (or apple cider) rather than water, to feed their starter for the initial four days. The level of acidity of the juice urges the proper micro-organisms to propagate. You just need to use it for the very first four days if you desire to attempt making use of juice instead of water. After day 4, feed your starter with flour as well as water. Don't use milk, sugar, or any type of ingredients aside from water and also flour to feed your starter. *(see the Pineapple Juice Solution by Debra Wink).

Fresh entire grain flour has approximately 200 times the micro-organisms * as white flour, so using some whole grain flour aids to get the starter fermenting. Rye flour or whole wheat flour are excellent choices to utilize in making your new starter.

Some bakers like to make use of all whole grain flour with no white flour. Entire grain flour soaks up much more water than white flour, so expect grain as a starter as an entire to be drier as well as include additional water if you feel it is too scorched (make use of a various hydration degree).

Your starter should have the consistency of a thick pancake batter or a muffin batter. With time, the fermentation procedure compromises the combination as well as the gluten is thinner and can have a layer of liquid on top (especially for higher hydration starters). That isn't a problem; just blend in the juice, pour out fifty percent of your starter, and also proceed to feed it.

When you prepare to use your mature starter, you will need to figure out just how much you will need to make your dough and change the quantity that you feed your starter as necessary.

The warmer you keep your sourdough starter, the more frequently you will certainly need to feed it Mother point you can do if you live in a sunny location is add a pinch of salt to reduce your starter down or change your ratio of starter to feed, pouring out even more of the starter as well as providing it more feed. Entire grain starters often require to be fed extra usually or a higher proportion of feed to the starter to maintain healthy and balanced given that they ferment extra quickly, you can additionally use a pinch of salt to aid control over fermenting.

MAKING YOUR OWN SOURDOUGH STARTER.

You can attempt your hand at making your sourdough starter. To maximize your chances of turning on an energetic starter, usage either component fresh ground whole grain flour or rye flour in your blend.

After the blend has begun to ferment, start to feed the mixture water and white flour (either All-Purpose or Bread flour), if you prefer a white sourdough starter. Or maintain feeding the mixture with wholegrain flours to have a whole grain starter. You could attempt something such as this.

The First Day: Add:

- V4 cup organic rye or wheat flour(freshly ground functions best).

- V4 mug bread flour.

- lh cup pineapple or apple cider (you can utilize pure water; however, it takes a couple of days much longer to obtain going).

Stir well to incorporate lots of oxygen and let the container of the flour/juice mixture sit, lightly covered, at area temperature level. There is a propensity in those just starting in sourdough cooking to maintain their starters and also doughs at hot temperatures to rush points up.

This is not continuously desirable, specifically for a sourdough starter. Attempt to preserve the new starter in a place that is in between 68-80F (20-26C) degrees. A higher temperature level encourages unfavorable micro-organisms in a brand-new starter that isn't yet steady adequate to ward off intruders. Organic flours produced without chemicals are more probable to get an excellent sourdough starter going.

The pineapple or apple cider is made use of for the acid conditions they offer, which motivate the wanted yeasts as well as bacteria and also dissuade the undesirable bacteria/yeasts. This was investigated by Debra Wink and even blogged about in her post "The Pineapple Juice Solution." This short article is readily available at BBGA.org for registered participants. This starter procedure was established in cooperation with Debra Wink as well as I am grateful for her experience.

Day Two: Stir, nothing else is required on day two.

Day Three:

Whether you see bubbles or otherwise, pour out fifty percent of your starter mix and also feed the starter with:

- 1/2 mug of pineapple juice or apple cider (or water) - 1/4 cup of rye or whole wheat flour.

- 1/4 cup of bread flour Pouring out half of the starter will undoubtedly give any type of yeasts or micro-organisms that exist, a more significant proportion of food as well as will undoubtedly water down for any kind of hostile bacteria.

Day Three and Four:

Follow the same feeding as in Day One and Day Three.

Day Five via day Fourteen.

Now each day for the following ten days, pour off fifty percent of your starter mixture and feed with 1/2 mug water (juice is no much longer necessary after day 4) as well as 1/2 mug flour mix. Now is the time to start if you want to have a white flour starter.

You are feeding the white starter flour rather than rye or whole wheat flours (making use of even more white flour at each feeding and much less wholegrain flour is much easier on the starter, as you are switching over flours, after a pair of days, use only white flour).

If you wish to have a rye or whole wheat starter, as opposed to feeding by volume(utilizing mug procedures), weigh the water and also rye or whole wheat flour and use equivalent weights of each ingredient to create a 100% hydration starter. An example would certainly be to possibly feed the starter with 2 oz of water as well as 2 oz of rye flour (or wheat flour. It takes about two weeks for your brand-new sourdough starter to come to be stable and also have the power needed to cook up great bread. During these two weeks, you will be working towards a regular starter and motivating the establishment of a symbiotic relationship between desirable bacteria (Lactobacilli) and also yeasts. A few of things that can trigger issues when trying to society a new starter are:

Old Flour - acquire high top quality, natural flours which are not also old or unhealthy, ideally natural.

Water - the chemicals in city water can be a trouble for starters, use fresh, filtered water or good well water.

Time and also Temperature - hold your horses; do not attempt to rush the procedure by maintaining the starter in a hot area (over 80 F) since a culture which is also cozy can motivate harmful germs to take control of.

Contamination- Be cautious regarding using a tidy spoon as well as a starting with a clean container to stay clear of harmful microorganisms contamination or go across corruption with another starter.

A word about hydration.

In bread cooking, hydration indicates the ratio of water to flour. A damp starter is around 166% hydration. A thicker starter is 100% hydration (which suggests that the water is 100% the weight of the flour).

Or one more example for a thicker starter would undoubtedly be to include 5 oz of flour and also 5 oz of water (for a starter that is 100% hydration). Make sure you have sufficient starter for your recipe and enough left over to maintain the starter going. An excellent proportion of feed to starter may be 1:1:1 or.5: 1: 1 with the very first number being the starter, the other, the water, and also the third the flour.

Steels can react with the acids in the starter as well as kill the starter or produce unfavorable tastes. You can use stainless spoons and bowls for blending dough, etc., but do not use a steel container for saving your sourdough starter.

Wood may hold the microbes in the fiber and also potentially infect if you make use of more than one starter.

If you do not wish to wait two weeks to see if you have an excellent starter or you have currently attempted and can not seem to obtain a good sourdough starter going, acquire a developed, stable sourdough starter from a neighbor or a sourdough starter with the web and also reactivate it.

Water and Flour:

Tap water alone is not high and can kill the starter straight-out or over time. Do not utilize bleach or soap to cleanse a sourdough starter container, usage only hot water. Newly ground flours are excellent for feeding a starter, yet age the flour for one to two weeks before making the dough if you grind it yourself.

KEEPING A STARTER HEALTHY

The older sourdough books which advise you to include active ingredients to your starter, like leftover dough, old biscuits,

If you want to experiment with your sourdough, just remove a small part and put it in another container to test without risking damaging your main product. Experimentation can be enjoyable, simply make sure to eliminate the starter you are experimenting with from the original starter as well as leave your initial starter alone. I directly choose starters fed with only flours and water (juice can be made use of the very first few days to obtain a starter going).

Not feeding the sourdough starter frequently or using the starter when it isn't sufficiently refreshed/fed is a prevalent issue, especially for those brand-new to sourdough baking.

I have tried numerous times to utilize a starter that smelled as well vinegary and was too far past its prime. I thought that including flour as well as water throughout mixing ought to be comparable to feeding the starter.

Feed your sourdough starter day-to-day if it is at room temperature level. If the starter scents acidic, put many of it out and develop it back up by feeding it a more significant proportion of flour/water before using it to make the dough.

A starter that is 166% hydration and also fed with a reduced proportion of feed to the starter will certainly not always look bubbly when it is all set to make use of; sometimes, it can seem dead. By a reduced proportion of feed to the starter, I imply that the quantity of the starter battery is above the amount of feed it gets. For example, if you have 2 cups of ripe starter, and also you feed it with one mug of water/flour blend, it will undoubtedly disappoint as much task as if you had one mug of ripe starter, and also you feed it with 2 cups of water/flour combination. It will undoubtedly astonish you at just how vigorous it is, even when it looks inactive. A very liquid starter fed with a considerable amount of feed may reveal a top layer of thin bubbles the morning after feeding. In contrast, the starter with a reduced amount of feed might disappoint any task.

When you feed it also cut off a quantity for too long of a time, it will, at some point, not be as active or healthy.

Starters can be impacted by bad water quality. The pastry shop across the bay from me had troubles for years with not being able to utilize the wild yeasts as a result of inadequate water high quality. I sent them several of my Northwest starters, and the first set passed away. I asked some concerns regarding the starter treatment and discovered they were making use of city faucet water to feed the starter and make the dough. City water has chlorine and various other chemicals in it that can be deadly to sourdough yeasts. The pastry shop has been effectively baking beautiful sourdough, considering that filtering their water.

Chlorine, there may be other chemicals in city tap water that can damage sourdough yeasts. Find the most excellent water you can as well as use it for both feeding the starter and for making up the dough. Filtering system water is generally excellent. Distilled water is not the best to use for sourdough, as it is free of mineral salts which are not useful and essential for nourishing yeasts and bacteria. Distilled water is still more helpful to unfiltered faucet water. If faucet water is all that is conveniently offered to you, boil the water, cool it, and afterward pour it into a container that you can maintain loosely covered. By doing this, some of the unpredictable gasses have a chance to dissipate. Leave the box, loosely covered for 24-- 48 hrs, then cover as well as save it for usage in feeding your starter and the blending of your dough. Using steamed faucet water has achieved success for those who just have faucet water readily available to them or if they don't understand what may be in the water, as in light or exclusive well water sources. I have heard that some individuals have not to worry about utilizing their faucet water with sourdough baking. Try a test using your tap water and feeding a percentage of sourdough starter, which you have allotted, and also check the results. The most recent starter I have dealt with in Hawaii would not even prosper after trying for two weeks. I was using city water. I finally threw it out and began another society making use of filtered catchment water (rainwater), the starter is doing quite possibly and also will make an excellent enhancement to my collection of sourdough beginners from all over the world.

Filthy rotten feet, vomit, harmful cheese are some of the summaries I have heard to define a starter with a nasty smell. A toxic smell can likewise happen when the proportion of feed to the starter is as well low (like not putting out or using any kind of starter and feeding just a tiny amount of water/flour). When reactivating a dehydrated starter, there can be a "bad" smell for a couple of days as it gets started, the smell should disappear, replaced by a terrific yeasty odor by day 5 or 6 with a reactivated starter.

To recoup a starter that looks or smells questionable, eliminate about 1/4 mug of the starter as well as it established aside in a tidy dish. Throw out the remainder of the starter and also tidy the starter container well, scratching down the sides and even cleaning with hot water.

-- 48 degrees is best) if the room temperatures are too cozy, then you won't have to feed it as common, mainly if you don't cook very typically.

If a starter is a horrible shade like pink, orange, or something truly unusual, you need to pour everything out and not take opportunities. A lot of neglected starters or a starter that has been polluted can be recovered using the approach over.

Always utilize an energetic starter that has been fed properly. During warmer climate, feed your starter extra commonly if it is maintained out at area temperature. When you decide to feed your starter, make sure to blend vigorously to aid incorporate plenty of oxygen, which is valuable in getting your starter going as well as keeping it healthy.

Note: It is not optimal to keep sourdough beginners in a refrigerator environment. Later on in this phase, the drawbacks of fridge storage space, where the temperature is maintained or below 40 degrees Fahrenheit, are reviewed.

PART TWO

SOURDOUGH BREAD & PIZZA RECIPES

WHITE SOURDOUGH

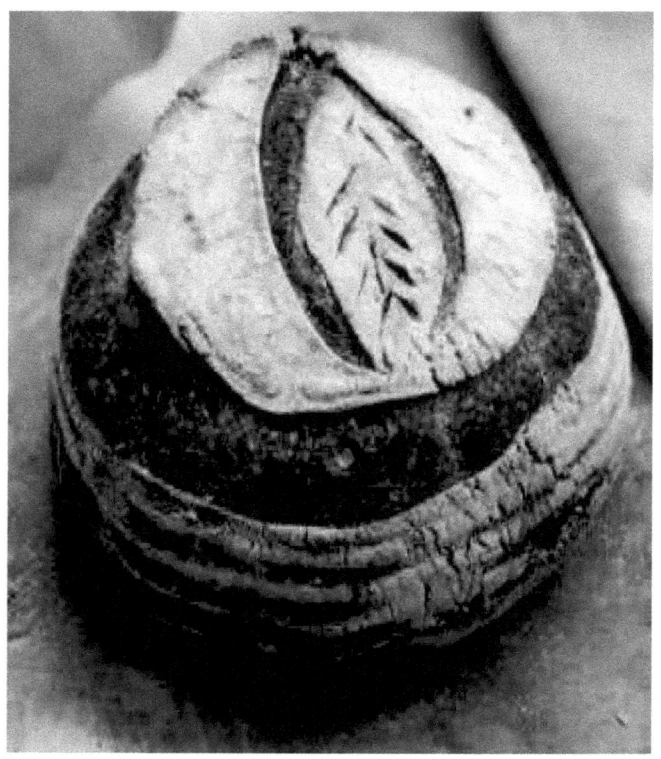

Ingredients

250 g / 2 cups healthy white bread 4
g / ¾ teaspoon salt
150 g / 150 ml / ⅔ cup of hot water
75g Starter White Dough Cup / Weld / Lift Dough Basket
(500g / 1lb Capacity) or Accessory
clean linen or tea/kitchen towel made from flour and flour
and baking oven (optional) parchment paper-lined baking
sheet

Prepare 1 Small Circle

1. Mix the flour and salt in a bowl (smaller). This is a dry mix (A)

2. In another (larger) mixing bowl, weigh the water and sourdough starter. Stir until it's well combined.
This is a wet mix. (B) (C)

3. Add the wet mix to the wet mix. Mix with a wooden spoon and later with your hands to form a dough. Use a plastic scraper to clean the side of the bowl and make sure everything is clean.
The ingredients are well mixed. (D) (E) (F)

4. Cover the container containing the dry mixture and allow it to rest for ten minutes.

5. After this, leave the dough in the bowl, remove the side part and press it in the middle. Rotate the container slightly and repeat the process with another portion of the dough.
Repeat eight more times.
The entire process should only take about 10 seconds, and the dough should hold up. (G) (H)

6. Cover the container again and allow it to rest for ten minutes.

7. Repeat steps 5 and 6 twice, and step 5 back. Cover the bowl and release it to rise for 1 hour. (I)

8. Gently wipe the clean work surface with flour.
Put the dough to the work surface. (J)

9. Form the dough into a smooth, rounded disk. (K) (L)

10. Expose the dough lifting/control basket or mat with clean bedding or a clean tea/kitchen towel. Sprinkle with flour and place the dough inside she. (M)

11. Now sprinkle the mixture with flour. (N)

12. Allow it to rise until it doubles in size; It will take 3-6 hours.

13. Preheat oven at 240 ° C (475 ° F gas) 9 for 20 minutes before baking.

Place the baking sheet on the bottom of the oven to preheat. Put water in the cup and set aside.

14. When the dough has doubled, remove it from the basket or accessories on the bread crust or prepared baking sheet. (OR)

15. Peel off the bedding or towel lightly. (Q)

16. Cut out circular patterns on the surface of the bread with a pair of sharp kitchen scissors. (Q)

17. Slide the dough into a preheated oven on a baking sheet or transfer it from the crust to a hot stone using a baking stone.

Pour the reserved cup of water inside the hot baking sheet and lower the oven temperature to 220 ° C (425 ° F) of gas 7.

18. Bake for about 30 minutes, or until it turns golden.

19. To make sure the bread is well baked, tilt it upside down and touch the bottom; It should sound hollow.

20. If you're not ready, return it to the oven for a few minutes. If you are prepared, place it on a wire rack to cool.

WHOLEGRAIN SOURDOUGH

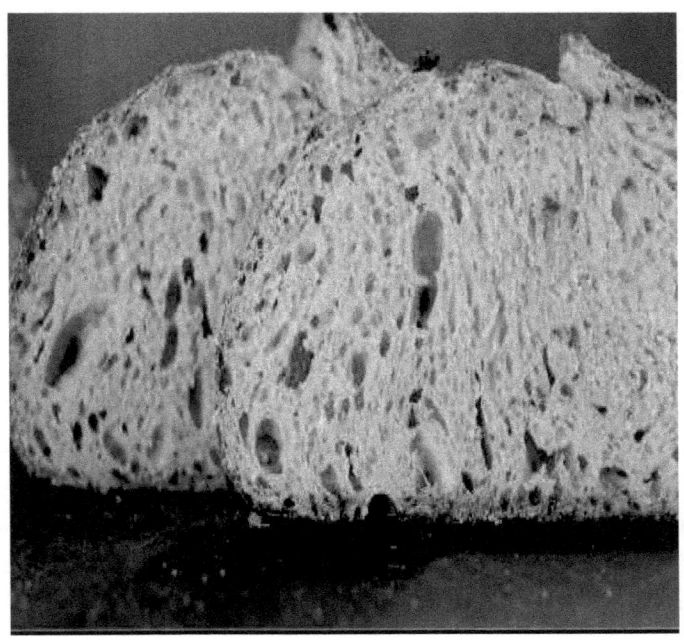

Ingredients

200 g / 1⅓ cup chopped/sliced wheat
200 g / 200 ml / 1 cup little hot water
400 g / 3¼ cup whole wheat / whole wheat flour 12
g / 2 teaspoons of salt
160 g / ⅔ cup white or whole wheat flour/sourdough at
least 140 g / 140 ml / ⅔ cup warm water
wheat-bran mix (see Suppliers & Stocks, page 173) long
hopper / dough hopper (900g / 2Lb capacity)
peeled bread crust and baking stone (optional)
baking sheet lined with parchment paper

Prepare 1 Big Circle

1. In a (smaller) mixing bowl, mix chopped/sliced wheat and 200 g / 1 cup of water and a low it to soak until softened.

2. In another (smaller) bowl, mix 400 g / 3¼ cups of flour and salt.

This is a dry mix.

3. In another (larger) mixing bowl, mix sourdough starter and 140 g / 140 ml // cup of water until well combined. Add the soaked wheat.

This is a wet mix.

4. Mix the dry and wet mixture until well combined.

Add water if the dough is too hard.

5. Cover the bowl containing the dry mix and let it steep for ten minutes.

6. After this, knead the dough as in step 5.

7. Cover the pan and allow it to sit for ten minutes.

8. Do steps 6 and 7 twice, then step 6 again.

Cover the bowl and let it rise for 1 hour.

9. Gently empty a clean work surface with a mixture of wheat and bran.

10 Place the dough on the work surface, roll with your hands to a mix, i.e., length and width of the check basket. (TO)

11. Sprinkle more wheat and bran mixture into the storage basket and put bread in it. (B)

12. Leave the dough to rise to twice its original size; this will take 3-6 hours. (C)

13. Preheat oven 20 minutes before baking 240 ° C (475 ° F) Gas 9.

Place the baking sheet at the bottom of the oven to preheat. Fill the cup with water and put it aside.

14. When the dough has doubled, transfer it from the crust to the crust of the bread or the prepared baking sheet. (D)

15. Slide the bread into a preheated oven on your baking sheet or, if you use a baking stone, transfer it from the crust to hot stone.

 Pour the cup of water set aside into the hot baking sheet and reduce the oven temperature to 220 ° C (425 ° F) of gas 7.

16. Bake for about 30 minutes, or until lightly browned.

17. To make sure the bread is baked, tilt it upside down and touch the bottom; It should sound hollow.

18. If you're not ready, return to the oven for a few minutes. If you are prepared, place it on a wire rack to cool.

LEVAIN DE CAMPAGNE' BREAD

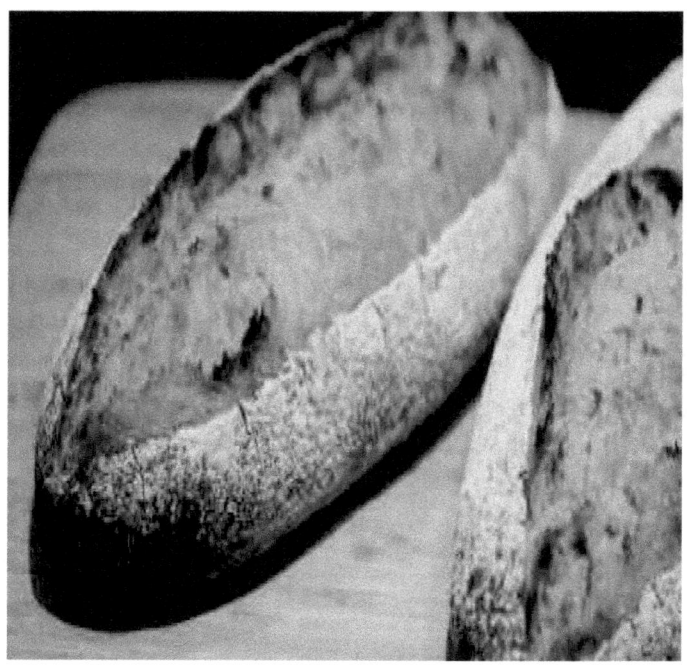

Ingredients

250 g / 2 cups healthy white bread

100 g / ¾ cup whole wheat flour / whole wheat flour 50

g / ½ rye / dark rye flour

6 g / 1 teaspoon of salt

150 g / start cups of white sourdough 300 g / 300 ml / 1¼ cups hot water round mass test/lift basket (900g / 2Lb capacity) peeled bread crust and baking stone (optional) baking sheet lined with parchment paper

Preparation

1. Mix the flour with salt in a bowl (smaller).

This is a dry mix (A)

2. In another (larger) mixing bowl, mix sourdough starter and water until well connected. This is a wet mix. (B)

3. Add the dry and wet mixture until its well mixed. The dough will be a little soft, but don't despair, and don't try to add more flour! (C) (D)

4. Cover the pan that contains the dry mix and let sit for ten minutes.

5. After ten minutes, press the dough as in step 5.

6. Cover the bowl again and let it sit for 10 minutes.

7. Apply steps 5 and 6 twice, then step 5 back.

8. Cover the container and allow it to rise for 1 hour.

9. Gently wipe the clean work surface with flour.

Put the dough to work surface and shape in a smooth, rounded disc. (AND)

10. Sprinkle the dough/hopper with flour.

 Put the mixture and sprinkle with flour. (F) (G)

11. Let the dough rise until it is twice its original size; this will take 3-6 hours. (H)

12. Preheat oven to 20 minutes before baking 240 ° C (475 ° F) Gas 9.

Place the baking sheet at the bottom of the oven to preheat.

Fill the cup with water and put it aside.

13. When the dough has risen to twice its original size, transfer it from the crust to the crust of the bread or the prepared baking sheet. (I J)

14 Using a sharp knife, cut a simple pattern on the surface of the dough. (K)

15. Slide the bread into a preheated oven on a baking sheet or transfer it from the crust to a hot stone using a baking stone.

Pour the reserved cup of water inside the hot baking sheet and lower the oven temperature to 220 ° C (425 ° F) of gas 7.

16. Bake for about 30 minutes, or until lightly browned.

17. To make sure the bread is baked, tilt it upside down and touch the bottom; It should sound hollow.

18 If you're not ready, put it back in the oven for a few minutes. If you are prepared, place it on a wire rack to cool.

WHITE WHEY SOURDOUGH

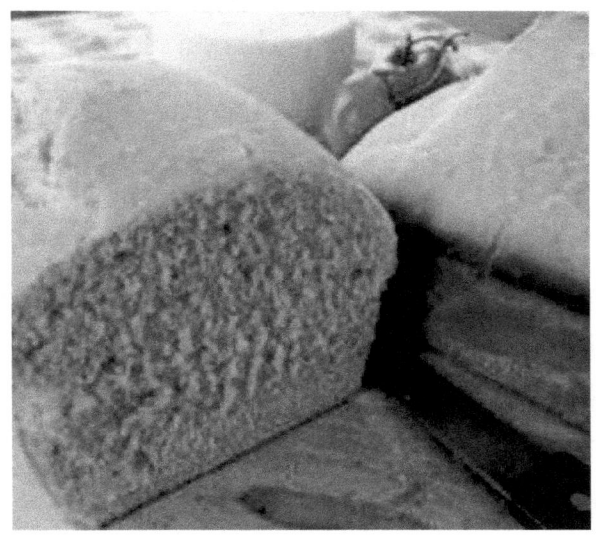

Ingredients

160 g / cups of white sourdough starter (see page 11) 300 g / 300 ml / 1¼ cup of serum (squeezed from

1 liter/liter of plain yogurt) or frothed milk 200 g / 1⅔ cup of strong white flour/bread

220 g / 1¾ cups of strong white bread 8

g / 1½ teaspoon salt

Welding basket for hive/dough (900g / 2lb capacity) or bedding for paper covers or pure tea/kitchen paper

peeled bread crust and baking stone (optional)

baking sheet lined with parchment paper

Preparation

1. In a mixing bowl (bigger), weigh the starter and buttermilk and mix with a wooden spoon until well mixed.

2 Add 200 g / 1⅔ cup flour and mix well.

This is advancement.

3. Cover and leave to ferment overnight in a cool place.

4. The next day, before fermentation, some bubbles should appear on the surface. (A)

5. In a mixing bowl (smaller), mix 220 g / 1¾ cup of flour and salt.

This is a dry mix.

6. Add dry mix to pre-ferment and mix until combined.

7. Cover with a container containing the dry mix.

8. Allow it to stand for ten minutes.

9. After ten minutes, knead the dough as in step 5.

10. Cover the bowl and let sit for another ten minutes.

11. Apply steps 9 and 10 twice, then step 9 again. (B)

12. Cover the pan and allow it to rise for 1 hour.

13. Gently wipe the clean work surface with flour.

Put the dough on the work surface.

14. Roll the dough into a smooth, rounded disk.

15. Align the dough control / lift basket or mat with a clean sheet or dishcloth. Sprinkle with flour and place the dough inside she. (C)

16. Let it grow until it doubles in size; It will take 3-6 hours. (D)

17. Preheat oven to 240 ° C for approximately 20 minutes before baking (475 ° F gas) 9.

 Place the baking sheet at the bottom of the oven to preheat.

Put water inside a cup and set aside.

18. When the dough has doubled, transfer it from the basket or cake to the bread crust or prepared baking sheet.

19. Peel off the bedding or towel lightly.

20. Cut a sheet of bread on the surface of the dough with a sharp, serrated tooth knife. (F)

21. Slide the dough into a preheated oven on a baking sheet or transfer it from the crust to a hot stone using a baking stone.

 Pour the reserved cup of water inside the hot baking sheet and lower the oven temperature to 220 ° C (425 ° F) of gas 7.

22. Bake for 30 minutes/ until golden.

23. To make sure the bread is baked, tilt it upside down and touch the bottom; It should sound hollow.

24. If you are not ready, return to the oven for a few minutes. If you are prepared, place it on a wire rack to cool.

SOURDOUGH GRISSINI

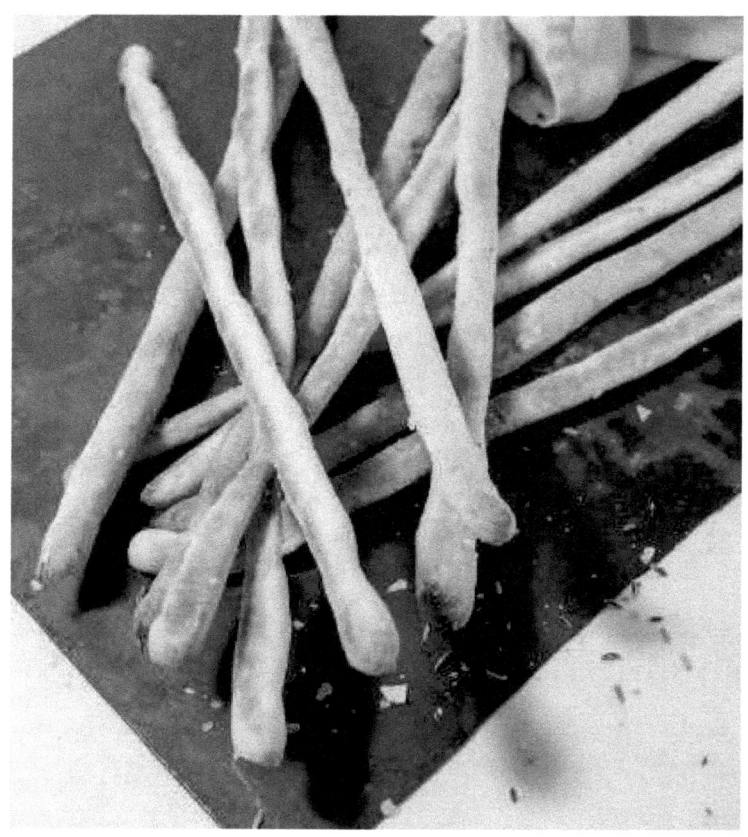

Ingredients

200 g / 1⅔ cup white/bread flour or Italian flour "oo." 4

g / ¾ teaspoon salt

100 g / cups white sourdough starter 110 g / 110 ml/cups low
to hot water

20 g / 20 ml / 1 tablespoon plus 1 teaspoon of olive oil

parchment paper-lined baking sheets

Preparation

1. Mix flour and salt in a bowl (smaller).

 This is a dry mix.

2. In another (larger) mixing bowl, mix sourdough starter and water until well combined. Add the olive oil. This is a wet mix.

3. Add the dry and wet mixture until it's well combined.

4. Cover the container containing the dry mix and allow it to steep for ten minutes.

5. After 10 minutes, knead the dough as in step 5.

6. Cover the bowl again and let it sit for ten minutes.

7. Do steps 5 and 6 twice again, then step 5 back.

8. Cover the pan and let it grow for 1 hour.

9. Gently wipe the clean work surface with flour.

 Put the dough on the work surface.

10. Slide the dough with your fingertips to flatten it and spread it out in a 5 mm / ¼ inch rectangle. (A)

11. Lightly cover with plastic wrap / plastic wrap and let sit for 15 minutes.

12. After 15 minutes, use a sharp knife to cut a rectangle of dough into 1 cm/inch. (B)

13. Stretch each grissini to spread and fold on the prepared baking sheets lightly. (C)

14. Leave in a cool place for 2 hours.

15. Before baking, preheat oven to 240 ° C (475 ° F gas) 9 for 20 minutes. Place the baking sheet on the bottom of the oven to preheat.

 Put water inside a cup and set aside.

16. Place the baking sheet in the preheated oven, pour a glass of water on the hot baking sheet, and reduce the oven temperature to 180 ° C (350 ° F) Gas 4.

17. Bake for about 20 minutes, or until it becomes golden brown.

18. Allow it to cool on cables.

POLENTA SOURDOUGH

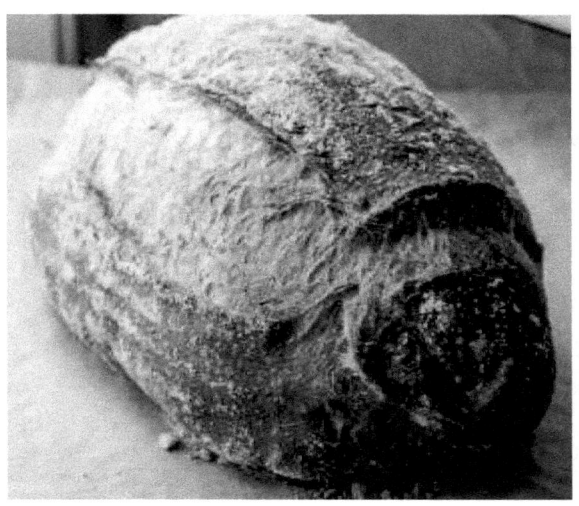

Ingredients

300 g / 2⅓ cups of strong white bread 8

g / 1½ teaspoon salt

60 g / ⅓ cup cornmeal or polenta 180

g / 180 ml / ⅔ cup of hot water

250 g / 1 cup white sourdough starter (see page 11) 2 teaspoons olive oil extra cornmeal / polenta, powdered

pastry basket (900 g / 2 lb. capacity) or flour crust with bread and baking stone (optional)

baking sheet lined with parchment paper Preparation

1. Mix the flour and salt in a container(smaller).

This is a dry mix.

2. Cook the cornmeal or polenta according to the producer's instructions. (A)

3. Turn the skillet off the heat and place a tablespoon of hot polenta in the mixing bowl (more giant).

 You need 150g of cooked polenta, so check the weight and remove the excess.

4. Add polenta water and stir. Be sure to do this while the polenta is still hot or warm and don't worry if there are a few small bumps:

This will add texture. (B)

5. In the polenta mixture, add the sourdough starter and olive oil and mix until well combined.

 This is a wet mix. (C)

 6. Add the dry and damp mixture by hand until combined.

7. Cover with a container containing the dry mix.

8. Allow it to stand for ten minutes.

9. After 10 minutes, knead the dough as in step 5.

10. Cover the bowl and let sit for another ten minutes.

11. Repeat steps 9 and 10 twice, then step 9 again. (D)

12. Cover the bowl and let it grow for 1 hour.

13. Lightly sprinkle a clean work surface with cornmeal or polenta. Put the dough on the work surface.

14. Form the dough into a smooth, rounded disk, covering it with whole cornmeal or polenta.

15. Sprinkle the powder/dough hopper with flour.

Put the mixture inside.

16. Allow the mixture to rise approximately twice the size; this will take 3-6 hours. (E)

 17. Preheat oven for 20 minutes before baking 240 ° C (475 ° F) Gas 9. Place the baking sheet at the bottom of the oven to preheat.

Fill the cup with water and put it aside.

18. When the dough has doubled, transfer it from the basket to bread crust or prepared baking sheet. (F) (G)

19. Using a sharp knife, cut parallel lines on the surface of the bread. (H)

20. Slide the dough into a preheated oven on a baking sheet, or if you use a baking stone, transfer it from the crust to the hot sand.

Pour the reserved cup of water onto the hot baking sheet and reduce the oven temperature to 220 ° C (425 ° F) of gas 7.

21. Bake for about 30 minutes /until golden.

22. To make sure the bread is baked, tilt it upside down and touch the bottom; It should sound hollow.

23. Mount it on the cooling cables.

TOMATO SOURDOUGH BREAD

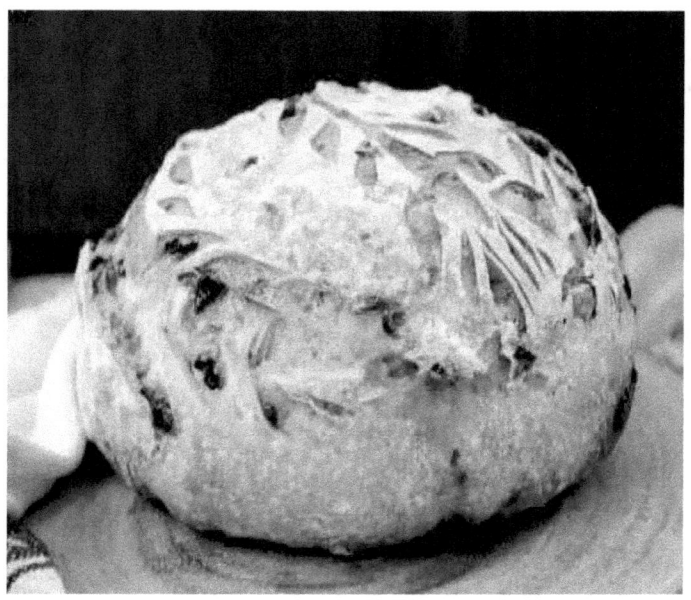

Ingredients

400 g / 3⅓ cups of healthy white bread

10 g / 2 teaspoons of salt

4 g / ¾ teaspoon celery seeds or ½ tablespoon freshly chopped rosemary leaves

 6 g / 1¼ teaspoons of nigella seeds (onion seeds) 40

g / 2½ tablespoons puree / pasta

200 g / 200 ml / ¾ cup of hot water

300 g / 1¼ cup white sourdough (see page 11) 2 teaspoons olive oil

long dough basket (900 g / 2 lb capacity) peeled

bread crust and baking stone (optional) baking

sheet lined with parchment paper

Preparation

1. Mix flour, salt, and seeds in a mixing bowl (smaller). This is a dry mix.

2. In another (larger) mixing bowl, mix tomato/water puree and water until well combined.

Add the entree with the sourdough. (A)

3. Add olive oil and stir.

This is a wet mix.

4. Mix the dry to the wet mixture until combined.

5. Cover the container where the mixture was dry

6. Allow it to stand for 10 minutes.

7. After ten minutes, squeeze the dough as in step 5.

8. Cover the bowl and let it sit for ten minutes.

9. Repeat steps 7 and 8 twice, then step 7 again.

10. Cover the pan and let it grow for 1 hour.

11. Gently wipe the clean work surface with flour. Place the dough on a work surface and shape it with your hands, in oatmeal, until it is approximately the length and width of your dough basket.

12. Pour the flour into the dough/roll basket and put the bread in it.

13. Allow the dough to rise approximately twice the size; this will take 3-6 hours. (B)

14. Preheat oven for about 20 minutes before baking

240 ° C (475 ° F) Gas 9. Place the baking sheet at the bottom of the oven to preheat.

Put water inside the cup and set aside.

15. When the dough has doubled, transfer it from the crust to a bread pan or prepared baking sheet.

16. With a sharp knife, cut a straight line in the middle of the bread. (C)

17. Slide the dough into a preheated oven on a baking sheet or transfer it from the crust to a hot stone using a baking stone. Pour the reserved cup of water onto the hot baking sheet and lower the oven temperature to 220 ° C (425 ° F) of gas 7.

18. Bake it for 30 minutes, or until golden.

19. To make sure the bread is baked, tilt it upside down and touch the bottom; It should sound hollow.

20. If you're not ready, return it to the oven for a few minutes. If you are prepared, place it on a wire rack to cool.

BEETROOT SOURDOUGH

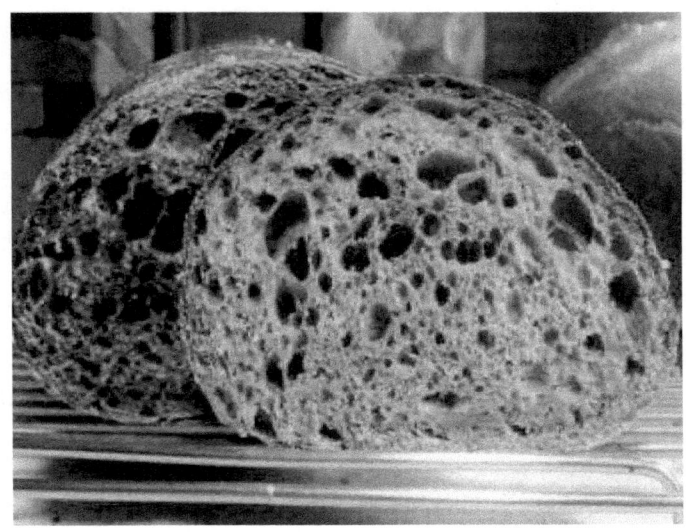

Ingredients

370 g / 3 cups white flour/bread flour 8

g / 1½ teaspoon salt

160 g / 5½ oz. Fresh raw beets/turnips, cleaned

220 g / 1 cup white sourdough (see page 11) 200 g / 200 ml / ¾ cup warm water

10 g / 2 teaspoons of olive oil

mass test / lift cart (900g / 2Lb capacity) (optional)

peeled bread crust and parchment paper-lined baking sheet.

Preparation

1. Mix the flour and salt in a smaller bowl.

This is a dry mix.

2. Peel the bread/beets and set aside. (TO)

3. Inside another (larger) mixing bowl, mix sourdough starter and water until well combined.

Now add the olive oil.

This is a wet mix.

4. Combine the dry and wet mixture and mix with hand until its well mixed, then add the ground beets/beets until well combined.

5. Cover the container containing the dry mix and let it steep for ten minutes.

6 Knead the dough as in step 5 after ten minutes.

7. Cover the bowl and allow it to sit for 10 minutes.

8. Do steps 6 and 7 twice again, then step 6 back. (B)

9. Cover the bowl and let it grow for 1 hour.

10. Gently wipe the clean work surface with flour.

Put the dough on the work surface.

11. Form the dough into a smooth, rounded disk.

12. Sprinkle the flour/dough hopper with flour. Put the dough and sprinkle with flour.

13. Allow the mixture to rise approximately twice the size; this will take 3-6 hours. (C)

14. Preheat oven 20 minutes before baking

240 ° C (475 ° F) Gas 9. Place the baking sheet at the bottom of the oven to preheat.

Put water in a cup and set it aside.

15. When the dough has doubled, transfer it from the crust to the crust of the bread / the prepared baking sheet. (D)

16. Slide the bread into a preheated oven on your baking sheet or, if you use a baking stone, transfer it from the crust to hot stone.

Pour the reserved cup of water onto the hot baking sheet and lower the oven temperature to 220 ° C (425 ° F) of gas 7.

17. Bake the bread for 30 minutes /golden brown.

18. To make sure the dough is baked, tilt it upside down and touch the bottom; It should sound hollow.

19. If you're not ready, return to the oven for a few minutes. If you are prepared, place it on a wire rack to cool.

SPICED CHEESE AND HERB SOURDOUGH

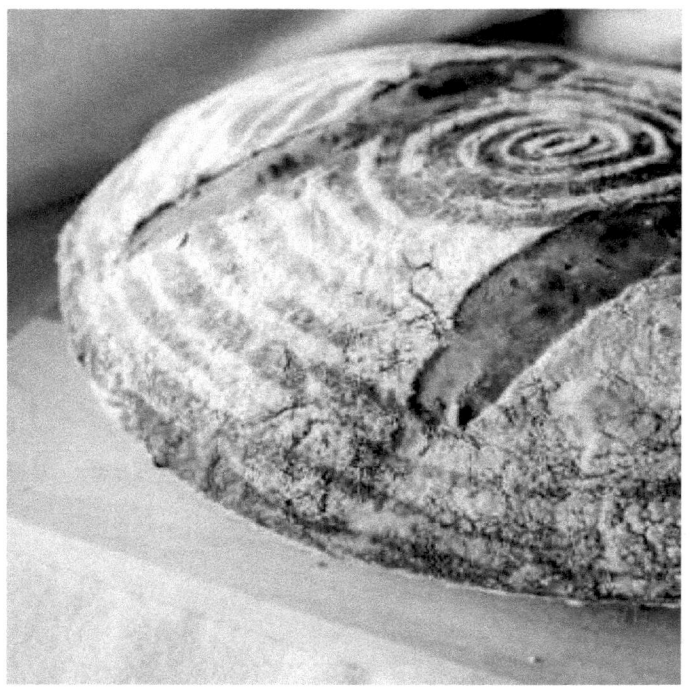

Ingredients

300g / 2½ cups of healthy white bread 8

g / 2 teaspoons of salt

2 g / ½ teaspoon ground chili powder or (hot peppers) flakes

150 g / 1½ cup grated cheddar cheese

Four tablespoons freshly chopped coriander/coriander or parsley

200 g / 1 cup white sourdough (see page 11) 180 g / 180 ml
/ ⅔ cup warm water

Four small baskets to test/lift the dough peeled

bread crust and baking stone (optional) baking

sheet lined with parchment paper

Prepare Four Mini Breads

1. In a (smaller) mixing bowl, mix flour, salt, and chili
powder or flakes.

This is a dry mix.

2. Mix cheese and herbs.

3. In another (larger) mixing bowl, mix sourdough starter
and water until well combined.

This is a wet mix.

4. Add the dry and curdled mix to the wet mix and mix by
hand until combined. (A)

5. Cover with a frying pan that had dry the mixture and let it
rest for ten minutes.

6. After ten minutes, knead the dough as in step 5.

7. Cover the bowl and allow it to sit for another ten
minutes.

8. Apply steps 6 and 7 twice, then step 6 again.

9. Cover the pan and allow it to rise for 1 hour.

10. Gently wipe the clean work surface with flour.

Put the dough on the work surface.

11. Divide the dough into four equal parts with a metal scraper or a sharp, serrated knife.

To be as precise as possible, weigh each piece and add or subtract the mass from the portions until they are all the same.

12. Form the dough pieces into smooth, rounded discs.

13. Sprinkle the powder/dough rolls with flour.

Put a piece of dough on each. (B)

14. Allow the mixture to rise for it to be as large as its initial size; this will take 3-6 hours.

15. Before baking, preheat oven to 240 ° C (475 ° F gas) 9 for 20 minutes. Place the baking sheet on the bottom of the oven to preheat.

Fill the cup with water and discard it.

16. When the dough has doubled its initial size, transfer it from the crust to the crust of the bread or the prepared baking sheet.

Using a sharp, serrated knife, cut curved cuts on the surface of the dough. (C)

17. Slide the bread into a preheated oven on a baking sheet or transfer from the crust to a hot stone using a baking stone.

Pour the reserved cup of water onto the hot baking sheet and lower the oven temperature to 220 ° C (425 ° F) of gas 7.

18. Bake for thirty minutes, or until golden.

19. To make sure the bread is baked, place a loaf upside down and touch the bottom; It should sound hollow.

20. If they're not ready, put them back in the oven for a few minutes. If you're ready, connect a cooling rack to the cables.

POTATO SOURDOUGH

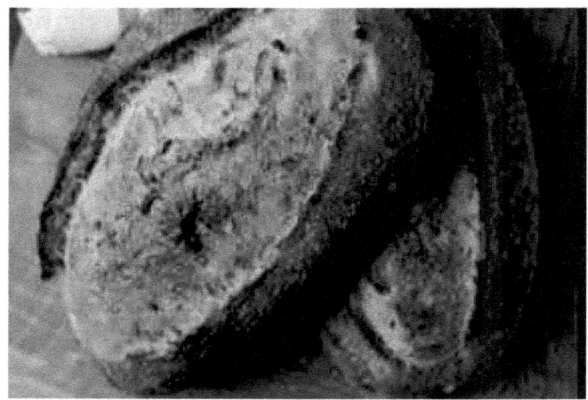

Potato bread is a form of bread in which potato flour or potatoes (raw or cooked) replace a portion of ordinary wheat flour.

Ingredients

250 g / 1 cup of starter with white sourdough (see page 11)
180 g / 180 ml / ⅔ cup of warm water

10 g / 2 teaspoons of olive oil

310 g / 2½ cups of healthy white bread 6

g / 1 teaspoon of salt

150 g / 5 oz. Peeled raw potatoes, skin grated or baked potatoes, broken into pieces to check/grow the basket (500g / 1lb capacity)

peeled bread crust and baking stone (optional)

baking sheet lined with parchment paper

Preparation

1. In a mixing bowl (bigger), mix the sourdough starter and water until well combined. Add the olive oil. This is a wet mix.

2. In another (smaller) mixing bowl, mix flour, salt, and potatoes.

This is a dry mix. (B)

3. Add the wet mix to the wet mix. (C)

4. Mix with your hands until combined. (D)

5. Cover the container containing the dry mix and let it steep for ten minutes.

6. After ten minutes, knead the dough as in step 5. (E)

7. Cover the container again and let it rest for 10 minutes.

8. Repeat steps 6 and 7 twice, then repeat step 6 back. (F)

9. Cover the bowl and let it rise for 1 hour.

10. Gently wipe the clean work surface with flour.

 Put the dough to the work surface and lightly sprinkle with flour. (G)

11. Form the dough into a smooth, rounded disk. (BOK)

12. Cover the dough/hopper with flour and place the dough inside. (J)

13. Allow the mixture to rise approximately twice the size; this will take 3-6 hours. (K)

14. Preheat oven for 20 minutes before baking

240 ° C (475 ° F) Gas 9.

Place the baking sheet at the bottom of the oven to preheat.

Put water inside the cup and set it aside.

15. When the dough has doubled, transfer it from the crust to a bread pan or prepared baking sheet. (L)

16. Slide the bread into a preheated oven on a baking sheet or transfer it from the crust to a hot stone using a baking stone.

Pour the reserved cup of water into the boiling water.

Bake and lower oven temperature to 220 ° C (425 ° F).

17. Bake for thirty minutes/ until golden. (M: Shows a loaf made of raw and grated potatoes and another made of baked potatoes.)

18. To make sure the bread is baked, flip it over and touch the bottom; It should sound hollow.

19. If you're not ready, return to the oven for a few minutes. If you are prepared, place it on a wire rack to cool.

FIG, WALNUT AND ANISE SOURDOUGH

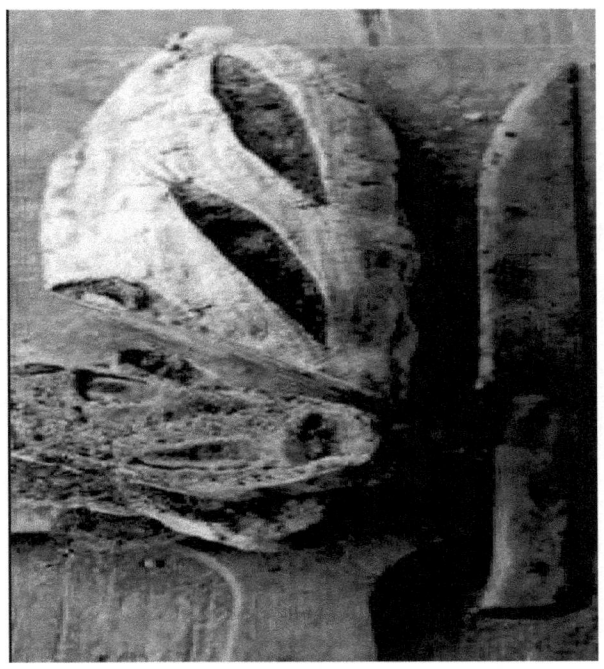

Fig and walnut are such an excellent combination, and the subtle addition of star anise is delightful. Try this bread to accompany the amorousness.

Ingredients

3 figs, chopped

40 g / ⅓ cup chopped walnuts 2

g / ½ teaspoon star anise

100 g / ¾ cup white flour/bread flour

45 g / ⅓ cup whole wheat flour / whole wheat flour

20 g / 2½ tablespoons dark rye / rye flour 3

g / ½ teaspoon of salt

65 g / cups of white sourdough starter 130 g / 130 ml / a cups of hot water

long dough basket (900 g / 2 lb capacity) peeled

bread crust and baking stone (optional) baking

sheet lined with parchment paper

Preparation

1. Mix the figs, walnuts and anise and reserve.

2. Mix the flour and salt in a container (smaller). This is a dry mix.

3. In the mixing bowl (bigger), mix the first sourdough and water until well combined.

This is a wet mix.

4. Add the dried and fig mixture to the wet mixture and stir until boiling is solidified

5. Cover the container containing the dry mix and let it steep for ten minutes.

6. After ten minutes, knead the dough as in step 5.

7. Cover the bowl and leave it to sit for ten minutes.

8. Apply steps 6 and 7 twice, then step 6 again.

Cover the pan and let it grow for 1 hour. (A)

9. When the dough has doubled in volume, tap it with your fist to release the air.

10. Gently wipe the clean work surface with flour. Transfer the ball of dough to the flour work surface.

11. Fold one edge of the dough toward the center.

Fold the opposite side over the middle. Now roll out the dough to make a sausage. The ends taper.

12. Sprinkle the flour/dough hopper with flour. Put the mixture inside. (B)

13. Let the dough rise until it is twice as large; this will take 3-6 hours.

14. Before baking, preheat oven to 240 ° C (475 ° F gas) 9 for 20 minutes.

Place the baking sheet on the bottom of the oven to preheat.

Fill the cup with water and put it aside.

15. When the dough has doubled, transfer it from the crust to a bread pan or prepared baking sheet.

Spread the flour on the bread. Using a sharp, serrated knife, cut diagonal lines across the surface. (C)

16. Slide the dough in a preheated oven inside a baking sheet, or if you use a baking stone, transfer it from the crust to hot stone.

Pour the reserved cup of water onto the hot baking sheet and lower the oven temperature to 220 ° C (425 ° F) of gas 7.

17. Bake for thirty minutes, or until golden.

Allow it to cool on the cables.

HAZELNUT AND CURRANT SOURDOUGH

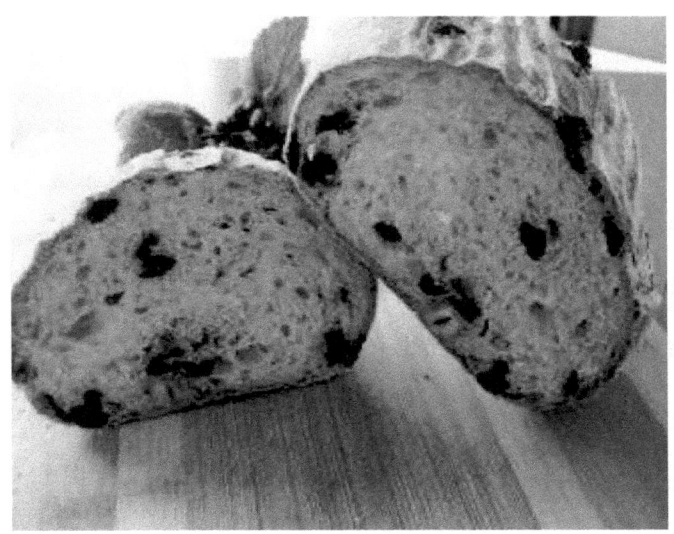

The most crucial aspect of this bread is the gently toasted hazelnuts. Toasting them brings out their flavor and complements the sweet currants. Try this bread with cheese.

Ingredients

120 g/1 cup lightly toasted hazelnuts, chopped 60

g/ 1/2 cup (Zante) currants

375 g/3 cups white healthy /bread flour

Six g/1 teaspoon salt

140 g/ 2/3 cup white sourdough starter

250 g/250 ml/1 cup of warm water

proofing/dough-rising basket (900-g/2-lb. capability) or colander proofing linen or clean tea/kitchen towel

floured bread peel and baking stone (optional).

Baking sheet lined with parchment paper

Preparation of 1 Large Loaf.

1. Mix the currants and nuts and set aside.

2. In one (smaller sized) mixing bowl, mix the flour and salt. This is the dry mixture.

3. In a (bigger) mixing bowl, blend the sourdough starter and water till well combined. This is the wet mixture.

4. Add the dry mix and nut mixture to the wet mixture and mix till it comes together.

5. Cover the bowl that had the dry mixture and leaves it for ten minutes.

6. Knead the dough as in Step 5 after ten minutes

7. Cover the bowl once again, and let go it for 10 minutes.

8. Repeat Steps 6 and 7 two times, then Step 6 back. (A).

9. Cover the container and allow it to rise for 1 hour.

10. Lightly dust a tidy work surface area with flour.

 Put the dough on the work surface area and shape it into a smooth, rounded disc.

11. Dough-rising basket or line a proofing, or a colander with proofing linen or a tidy tea/kitchen towel.

Dust freely with flour and lay the dough inside it.

12. Let rise till about double the size; this will take in between 3 and 6 hours. (B)

13. Before baking, preheat the oven to 240 ° C(475 ° F)Gas 9 for 20 minutes.

Place a roasting pan beneath the oven to pre-heat.

Fill a cup with water and set it aside.

14. When the dough has doubled in volume, suggestion it out of the basket or colander onto the bread peel or ready baking sheet. Carefully peel away the linen or towel. (C) (D)

15. Slash simple lines on the surface of the bread using a sharp, serrated knife.

16. Slide the dough into the preheated oven on its flat pan, or if using a baking stone, slide it from the peel onto the hot sand.

 Pour the reserved cupful of water inside the hot roasting pan and reduce the oven temperature to 220 ° C (425 ° F) Gas 7.

17. Bake for thirty minutes, or until golden.

18. To check if the bread is well baked, tip it upside down and tap the bottom-- it must sound hollow.

19. If it is not done, return it to the oven for some minutes. Set it on a wire rack to cool if it is done.

CHOCOLATE AND CURRANT SOURDOUGH

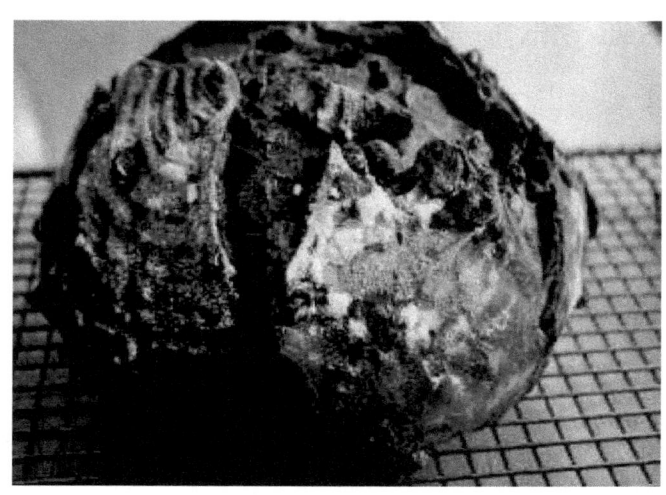

Ingredients

200 g / 1⅓ cup redcurrant (Zante)

80 g / ⅔ cup milk / semi-sweet chocolate chips

330 g / 2⅔ cups of healthy white bread

8 g / 1½ teaspoon salt

20 g / 2½ tablespoons cocoa powder

170 g / start cups of white sourdough (see page 11) 250 g / 250 ml / 1 cup of warm water

long dough basket (900 g / 2 lb capacity) peeled

bread crust and baking stone (optional) baking

sheet lined with parchment paper

Preparation

1. Mix the raisins and the chocolate and reserve.

2. Mix the flour, salt, and cocoa powder in a mixing bowl (smaller). This is a dry mix.

3. In the mixing bowl (bigger), mix the first sourdough and water until it is well mixed.

 This is a wet mix.

4. Add the dry and chocolate mixture to the wet mixture and mix until combined.

5. Cover the container containing the dry mix and let it steep for ten minutes.

6. After ten minutes, knead the dough as in step 5.

7. Cover the bowl and leave it to sit for ten minutes.

8. Apply steps 6 and 7 twice, then step 6 again.

Cover the pan and let it rise for 1 hour. (A)

9. When the dough has doubled in volume, tap it with your fist to release the air.

10. Gently wipe the clean work surface with flour. Transfer the ball of dough to the flour work surface.

11. Divide the dough into two; equal parts then roll each into a ball.

12. Sprinkle the flour/dough hopper with flour. Place two dumplings next to each other, so they sit together. (B)

13. Allow the dough to rise until it is twice as large; this will take 3-6 hours.

14. Preheat oven to 240 ° C (475 ° F gas) 9 for 20 minutes before baking.

Place the baking sheet on the bottom of the oven to preheat.

Fill the cup with water and set it aside.

15. When the dough has doubled, transfer it from the crust to a bread pan or prepared baking sheet.

Spread the flour on the bread. Using a sharp, serrated blade on the surface, cross the cross on the surface. (C) 16. Slide the dough in a preheated oven onto a baking sheet, or if you use a baking stone, transfer it from the crust to hot sand.

Pour a reserved cup of water in a hot baking sheet and lower the oven temperature to 220 ° C (425 ° F) Gas 7.

17. Bake for thirty minutes, or until golden.

18. To make sure the bread is baked, tilt it upside down and touch the bottom; It should sound hollow.

Allow it to cool on the cables.

CARAWAY RYE SOURDOUGH

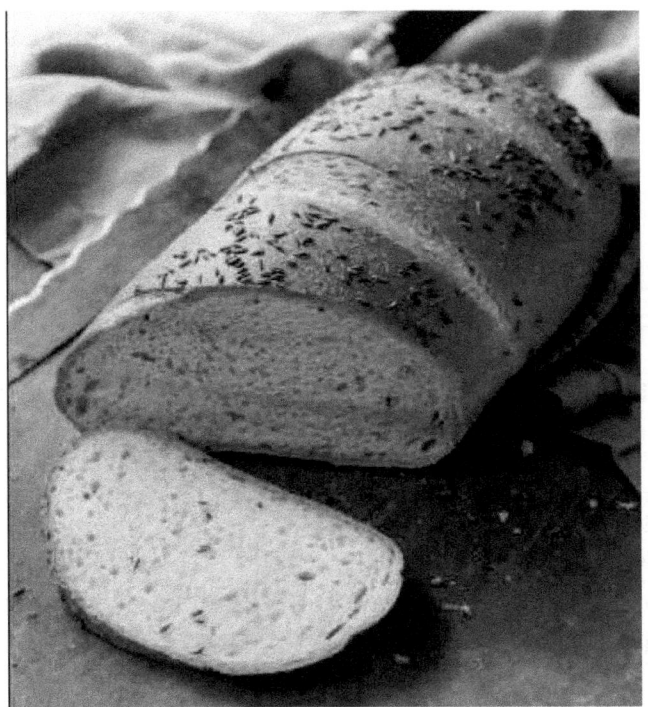

This is the classic type of rye bread found in Germany, with a slight hint of cumin. It looks incredible when baked because the crust breaks dramatically.

Ingredients

350 g / 3 cups rye flour / whole grain rye bread 150

g / 1½ cup of white bread

10 g / 2 teaspoons of salt

3 g / 1 teaspoonful of cumin seeds

250 g / 1 cup of rye acid starter (see page 11) 400 g / 400 ml / 1½ cup of hot water

pastry basket (900 g / 2 lb. capacity) flour and baking stone (optional) baking tray lined with parchment paper

Prepare 1 Big Circle

1. Mix flour, salt, and seeds in a mixing bowl (smaller). It

is a dry mix. (TO)

2. In another (larger) mixing bowl, mix sourdough starter and water until well combined.

This is a wet mix. (B)

3. Add the dry mix to the wet mix and stir until smooth and looks like a full suspension. (C) (D) 4 Cover the skillet containing the dry mix and let stand for 1 hour.

5. After 1 hour, transfer the dough to light, coarse flour on a platter.

6. Sprinkle more powder with dark rye/rye flour.

7. Roll the mixture into the flour.

8 Sprinkle the powder/dough hopper with flour. Put the dough inside and sprinkle with flour. (F) (G)

9. Allow the mixture to rise until it doubles; this will take 3-6 hours. (H)

10. Preheat oven to 20 minutes before baking

240 ° C (475 ° F) Gas 9.

Put the baking sheet at the bottom of the oven to preheat.

Put water inside a cup and set it aside.

11. When the dough has doubled its initial size, transfer it from the crust to the crust of the bread or the prepared baking sheet. (I)

12. Slide the dough into a preheated oven on a baking sheet or transfer it from the crust to a hot stone using a baking stone.

Pour the reserved cup of water onto the hot baking sheet and reduce the oven temperature to 230 ° C (450 ° F) Gas 8.

13. Bake for thirty minutes, or until lightly browned.

14. To make sure the bread is baked, tilt it upside down and touch the bottom; It should sound hollow.

15. If you're not ready, return to the oven for a few minutes. If you are prepared, place it on a wire rack to cool.

3-GRAIN BREAD

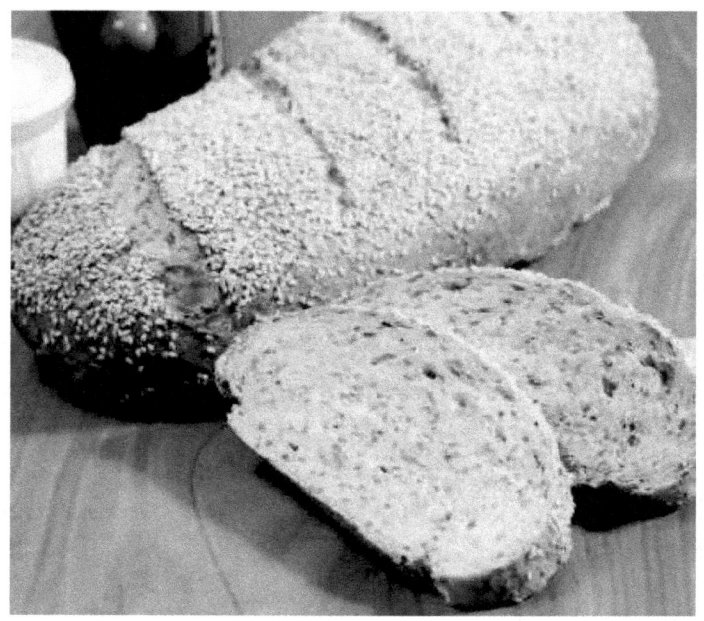

Ingredients

Two tablespoons fennel and coriander seeds, plus one tablespoon cumin seeds, for a 100 g / 100 ml / ½ cup cold water spice mix

50 g / ⅓ cup sunflower seeds 30 g

/ ⅓ cup flaxseed / flaxseed

12 g / 2 tablespoons porridge / old fashioned tooth 12

g / 2 tablespoons chopped / sliced wheat

180 g / ¾ cup rye acid starter (see page 11) 150 g / 150 ml / ⅔ cup hot water

250 g / 2 cups light rye flour

150 g / 1¼ cup of white bread 8

g / 1½ teaspoon salt

4 g fresh yeast or two g / ½ teaspoon dry/active dry yeast

50 g / 50 ml / 3 tablespoons of warm water

long dough basket (900 g / 2 lb capacity) peeled

bread crust and baking stone (optional) baking

sheet lined with parchment paper **Prepare 1**

Big Circle

1. To make the seasoning, mix the fennel, coriander, and cumin seeds and toast in a dry saucepan over low heat until the seeds are browned.

Allow it to cool, then grind with a grinder and mortar or spice mill.

2. Place 100 g / 100 ml / ½ cup water, sunflower seeds, flax/flaxseed, oats, and chopped/split wheat in a large bowl (mixing bowl) and mix. This is a wet mix. Cover and leave overnight in a cool place.

3. Simultaneously in another (bigger) mixing bowl, mix the sourdough starter and 150g / 150ml / Alice of warm water until well combined. Add rye flour lightly and mix the pasta.

Cover and leave it to ferment in a cool place throughout the night.

4. In the (smaller) mixing bowl the next day, mix the white flour, salt, and 1 tsp of the spices. This is a dry mix.

5. In a (smaller) bowl, melt the yeast in warm 50 g / 50 ml / 3 tablespoons water, then add it to the sourdough mixture and mix well.

6. Now mix the wet and dry mix until everything is combined.

The dough should be quite stiff and sticky, but if it seems too dry, add a little water.

7. Cover the container containing the dry mix and let it steep for 10 minutes.

8. Knead the dough as in step 5 after ten minutes. It will be pretty sticky

9. Cover the bowl and leave it to sit for ten minutes.

10. Do steps 8 and 9 twice, then step 8 again.

11. Cover the bowl and let it rise for 1 hour. (B)

12. Lightly dust the clean work surface of the oats. Transfer the dumpling to the desk (C)

13. Shape it with your hands, in oatmeal, until it is approximately the length and width of your payment basket. (D)

14. Sprinkle more oatmeal in the bowl and put the bread in it.

15. Allow the dough to rise approximately twice the size: 1- 2 hours. (E)

16. About 20 minutes before baking, preheat oven to 240 ° C (475 ° F gas) 9. Place the baking sheet on the bottom of the oven to preheat. Fill the cup with water and set aside.

17 When the dough has doubled, transfer it from the crust to a bread pan or prepared baking sheet.

Using a sharp knife, zig-zag around the surface. (F)

18. Slide the bread in a preheated oven onto a baking sheet or, if you use a baking stone, transfer it from the crust to hot stone.

Pour the reserved cup of water onto the hot baking sheet and lower the oven temperature to 220 ° C (425 ° F) of gas 7.

19. Bake for about 30 minutes, or until golden.

20. Allow it to cool on cables.

SEMOLINA BREAD

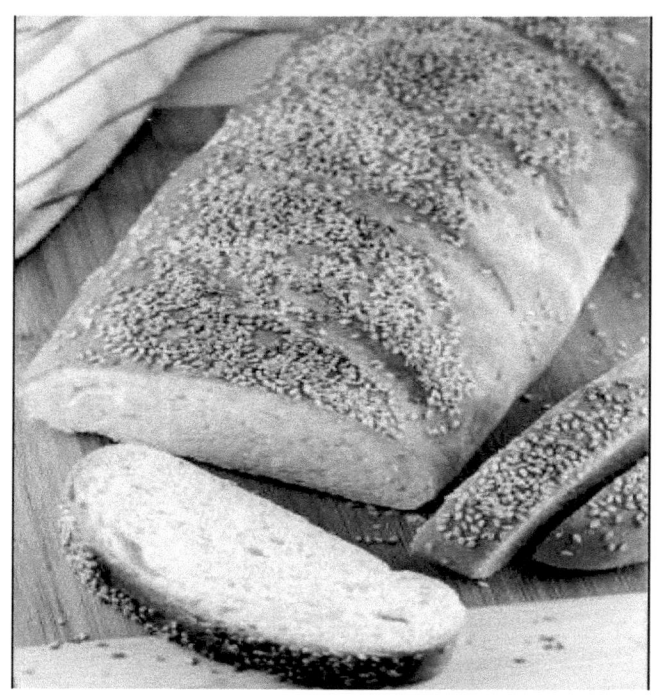

Ingredients

125 g / 1 cup white flour/bread flour or Italian flour "00" 3

g / ½ teaspoon of salt

25 g / 2 tablespoons white sourdough 150 g / 150 ml / ⅔ cup warm water

150 g / 1 cup plus two tablespoons of porridge

3 g fresh yeast or two g / ¾ teaspoon dry/active dry yeast 50

g / 50 ml / 3 tablespoons of warm water

5 g / 1 teaspoon of olive oil 15 g

/ 3 teaspoons of olive oil

baking sheet lined with parchment paper

Preparation

1. Mix both flour and salt in a smaller bowl. This is a dry mix.

2. In a mixing bowl (bigger), weigh the sourdough starter, 150g / 150 ml / ⅔ cup of water, and puree. (TO)

3. Mix with a wooden spoon until its well mixed. (B)

4. Cover and leave to ferment for 2 hours or overnight in a cool place.

This is fermented before (C)

5. When fermentation is complete, in the mixing bowl (bigger), dissolve the yeast in 50 g / 50 ml / 3 tablespoons of water and mix 5 g / 1 teaspoons olive oil (D)

6. Mix the yeast solution in the fermentation.

 This is a wet mix.

7. Add the wet mix to the wet mix. (AND)

8. Mix with a wooden spoon until combined. (F)

9. Cover and allow it to sit for 10 minutes. It will be very smooth at this stage.

10. Pour half of a 15 g / 3 tablespoons olive oil into another large bowl.

11. Using a dough scraper, shake the dough in a pan of olive oil. (G)

12. Pull the mixture to one side and press it in the center.

Rotate the bowl slightly and repeat the process with another portion of the dough.

Repeat the process twice. (H)

13. Allow it to stand for 10 minutes. (I)

14. Repeat steps 12 and 13 3 more times, adding the rest of the olive oil to prevent the pasta from sticking to the bowl. (J)

15. Let stand for 10 minutes.

16. Gently wipe the clean work surface with flour.

Put the dough on the work surface.

17. Fold the dough as in step 12 twice. (K) (L) (M)

18. Let it stand for 15-20 minutes.

19. After 15-20 minutes, fold the dough again, turning it to make a circle.

Flip it over and wrap it around any edge for a smooth, even feel the ball. (N)

20. Grease the prepared baking sheet with a shadow and place the dough on it.

Roll out the dough with a bite. (OR)

21. Using your fingers, poke a hole in the middle of the dough, then gently pull the side out until it turns into a ring. (P)

22. Allow it to rise for thirty minutes or until bubbles begin to form on the surface of the dough.

23. About 20 minutes before baking, preheat oven to 240 ° C (475 ° F gas) 9.

Place the baking sheet on the bottom of the oven to preheat.

Fill the cup with water and set it aside.

24. When the bread is ready to bake, sharpen with three knives on a 3-line surface. (Q)

25. Slide the dough into the preheated oven.

Pour the reserved cup of water onto the hot baking sheet and lower the oven temperature to 220 ° C (425 ° F) of gas 7.

26. Bake it for 35 minutes, or until golden brown. (R)

27. To make sure the bread is baked, tip it upside down and touch the bottom; It should sound hollow.

28. If you're not ready, return to the oven for a few minutes. If you are prepared, place it on a wire rack to cool.

PIZZA

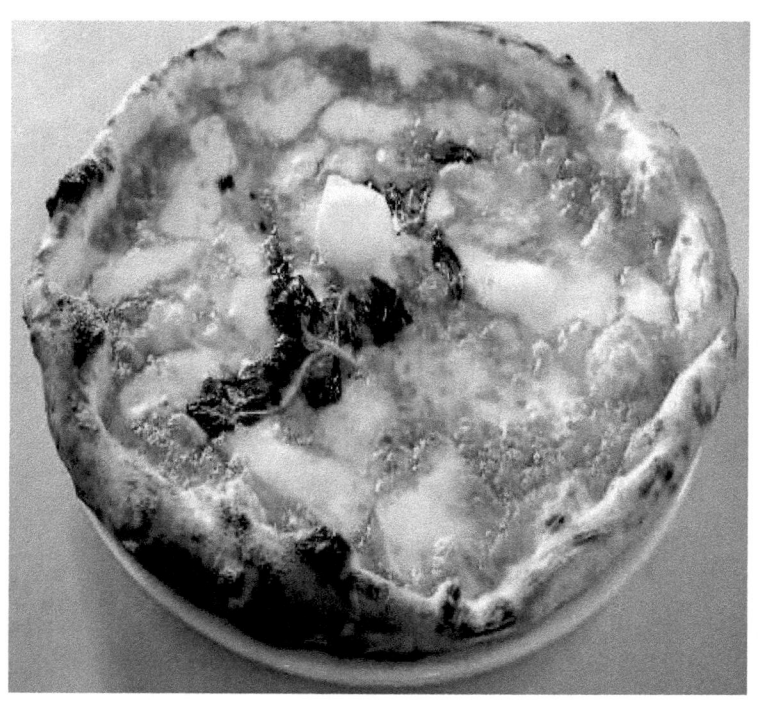

Sourdough Pizza Crust

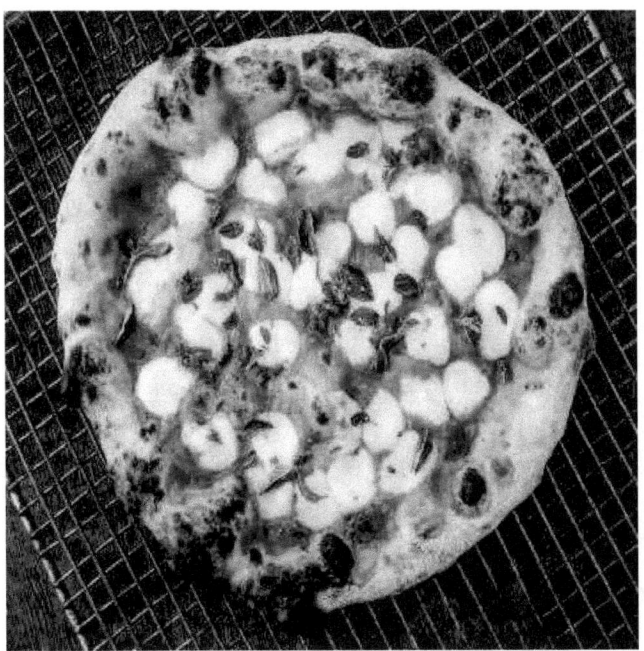

Pizza crust

Sauce bakers are always looking for creative ways to use an unnecessary starter. In the case of this pizza dough, the open crumbs and the characteristic sourdough flavors combine well with the daring ingredients and well-aged cheeses.

Preparation

10 minutes

Oven

16 to 18 min Total

4 hours 56 min

Performance

A 14-thick round or sizeable thick crust pizza; or two 12 "round thin-crust pizzas.

Pizza crust

Ingredients

1 cup (241 g) acid starter, uncleaned / discarded

1/2 cup (113 g) warm water

2 1/2 cups (298 g) King Arthur gluten-free universal flour

One teaspoon salt

1/2 teaspoon of instant or active dry yeast

Four teaspoons of pizza dough to taste, optional but delicious

Instructions

Insert any liquid into the top of the cooled starter before weighing 1 cup (241 g) in a large mixing bowl. Note: This is an excellent opportunity to add the rest of your launcher as needed.

Add warm water, flour, salt, yeast, and pizza dough aroma (if used).

Stir to combine, then knead for 7 minutes in a mixer with a dough hook until the dough loops around the hook and clears the sides of the bowl.

Place the dough in an oiled skillet, cover, and allow to rise to almost double.

Depending on the vitality of its initiator, it will take between two and four hours. For faster growth, place the dough in a warm place or double the yeast.

For two thin-crust pizzas, divide the crust in half and form each into a flattened platter.

Drain two 12 "olive oil pizza balls and brush the bottom with a brush.

Place the dough in the pans, cover, and let sit for 15 minutes.

After the rest, gently press the dough towards the edges of the pans before proceeding

Erin's Sourdough Pizza

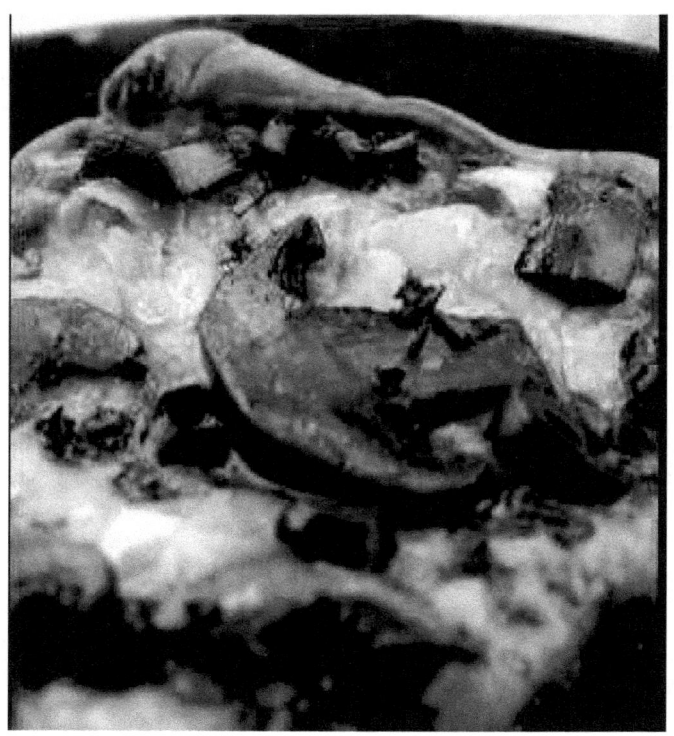

Ingredients

1 1/2 cups sour starter click here for free instructions 1

1/2 tablespoons coconut or olive oil

sea salt about 1 tsp

1 to 1 1/2 cups flour of your choice

optional meats, cheese, vegetables, etc.

Instructions

Would you like your pizza in the morning?

Pour starter, oil, and salt into a medium bowl and mix. After then add one cup of flour to the mixture and stir well. Then sprinkle a little flour on the counter.

Cover the dough mixture and start kneading.

Add flour as required.

Then knead the dough until all the ingredients are well combined.

Remember, you are looking for a mixture that is soft and not sticky.

If you see that your dough is too moist, add more flour. If it is too dry, add more water, starter, or whey to have a perfect mixture.

Once the batter is ready, return the dough ball to the bowl (lightly greased), cover with a plate, and cook overnight.

Or

Let the mixture sit for 30 minutes, then roll out and simmer like a greasy crust ready to grow.

Be sure to cover it with plastic wrap to prevent it from drying out. (Don't resort to aluminum foil!)

Once it's time to bake pizza.

Preheat oven to 450 degrees Fahrenheit or hotter for pre-baking. (If you have a pizza stone, preheat it here!)

While the oven is preheating, if you have not done so already, roll out the dough.

Knead the broken dough several times with a fork.

Then bake in the oven for about 5 minutes carefully. Don't let it get too dark.

This is just precooking.

Remove the pizza from the oven.

Chill and freeze for instant baking

Oregon

Cover with olive oil and add your favorite ingredients!

Bake your decorated sourdough pizza for 10 to 25 minutes, depending on oven temperature, ingredients, and thickness of the crust.

Enjoy!

Prescription Notes

* With my appetizer, I eat the night before morning to prepare the pizza dough. This ensures that I will have enough happy preparations to make myself and something left over for future sourdough adventures.

* I generally give the starter a sour ratio in a ratio close to 1: 1 (flour/water). Depending on what I do, I can use more flour for a thicker snack. It doesn't matter how you feed your motor for this recipe. It will correct any inconsistency while mixing.

* This recipe will work on a thick or thin crust. What is your wish? Roll out the dough accordingly.

* I like the second oven directly on top of the oven (I can reduce the heat depending on the amount of dressing).

This creates a delicious crispy crust. Because the coating is precooked, it is easy to peel it off the cookie jar and place it on the oven rack. Once the pizza is done, I slide it back onto the cookie sheet for easy cutting.

Slo-Mo Sourdough Pizza

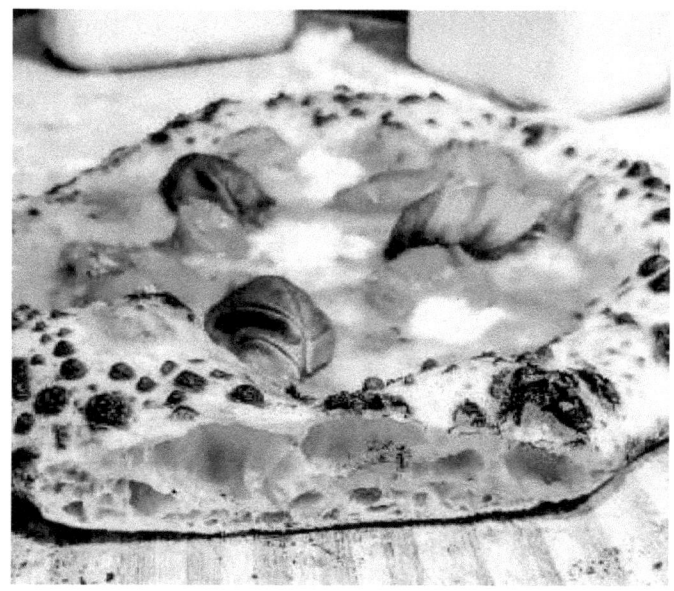

(A) Hydration 167 (67%)

Ingredients

280 g of pizza flour

25 g Levain 3-4 times fed as described in the recipe below

185 g of water

7 g of salt

Instructions

Levain

3-4 times fed: for the last feeding (to make your yeast) apply a ratio of 1: 2: 2 (Starter: Flour: Water).

The calculation is easy; you only need to finish the whole sourdough, as required in the recipe (in this case 25 g, so you need 5 g of starter, 10 g of flour and 10 g of water) Use your sourdough to reach maximum ages 4 to 5 hours (let it rise to room temperature 25 to 27 degrees Fahrenheit). This time frame is confusing and depends on the activity of your sourdough culture. I highly recommend that you use the same flour to build yeast as you use it for your regular sourdough diet.

(B) Autolyze
Ingredients

280 g of pizza flour (alternative: flour)

155 g of water

Levain 25g

7g of salt

30g of water (cold)

Instructions

Mix the flour and the required quantity of water and let the dough cover well for 2 hours at room temperature (Autolyze).

Add sourdough to the autolyzed dough and start kneading with the kitchen machine on low speed until the dough comes out of the bowl.

Continue kneading at a higher rate for 4-5 minutes and add the remaining water step by step.

Add salt along with the last bit of water.

Stop mixing after all the gluten has developed entirely (the temperature of the dough should not exceed 25-27 degrees Celsius).

Place the dough in a greased pan and let it ferment well for 45 minutes at room temperature of 25 degrees Fahrenheit.

Moisten the work surface with water, release the dough to the surface, and cover the mixture (follow the instructions in the Basics section: Basics | Open Crumbs - Batch of Sourdough | Laminate).

Return the dough to a greased skillet and let sit for 45 minutes.

Give the mixture a little fold and let it rest until the initial volume increases by about 40%.

After another slight fold, allow the dough to rest well in the refrigerator for 48 hours (5 degrees Fahrenheit).

The final test

On the day of pizza cooking, allow the mixture to acclimate for 120 minutes, place it on a moistened work surface, and divide it into two equal parts (245g each). Now, under tension (but without degassing), form balls and leave them covered (with the sealed side down) for 2-3 hours.

Oven

Heat oven and baking stone for at last half an hour

To shape the pizzas, sprinkle flour on the work surface and dumplings and place them on the floor.

 The next time, with your fingers, press all the air to form the center out. Once all the wind is in the edges, sift the hand outside and place the dough on the handles. Now gently roll the pizza to the desired size. The only thing he misses is the topping you want, so your pizzas are ready to bake (5-12 minutes depending on the temperature of your oven). If you have a pizza oven, it reaches at least 400 degrees Celsius; your pizzas will bake in 90-120 seconds.)

The previous recipe is equivalent to 2,245 g of pizzas.

Depending on the pizza flour you use, you can increase the hydration of the dough (the amount of water used in the main dough) and the fermentation time in your refrigerator.

Levain's assembly schedule – Example:

Because most of you keep a few days in the refrigerator during the day, your sour foods must be fed 3-4 times before buying yeast (the last feeding) for a scheduled cook. These supplements will reduce the acid load and increase the activity level of your motor.

For feeding, only work with minimal amounts of flour and according to the initial proportions (sourdough you have stored or the resulting number of the scheduled steps, such as those shown below) of flour and water. All the discarding produced can be ideally used to make an aromatic Levain flower. Here is a guide with instructions.

Friday morning: 1: 3: 3 (2 g inlet: 10 g of flour: 10 g of water)

Friday noon/afternoon: 1: 5: 5 (2 g of the previous phase: 10 g of flour: 10 g of water)

Friday night: 1:10:10 (2 g of the last stage: 20 g of flour: 20 g of water)

Saturday morning: LEVAIN: 1: 2: 2 (previous phase: flour: water): you must finish the total amount indicated in the recipe

This example will show you how you can plan your feeds. Look at the sourdough and try to estimate the time it will take to reach the peak at a specific feeding ratio. On a baking day, you will waste your yeast on the young side (4- 5 hours young at its peak). This also benefits from open crumbs and overheating.

Perfect Homemade Hand-Tossed Sourdough Pizza

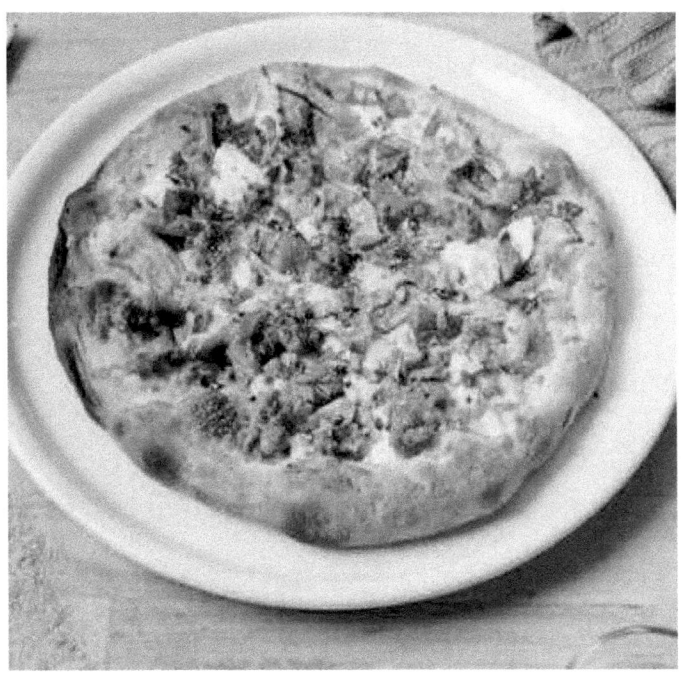

It's great! With Red Star Yeast and learn master pizzaiolo techniques on how to make the ideal homemade sourdough pizza with your hand.

Red Star Yeast Red Yeast - Skip the best entrees and use this yeast for authentic acid cultivation with the convenience of yeast!

Ingredients

450 grams of Neapolitan bread or flour 00

250 grams of water (cold or at room temperature)

One package (18 grams) of Red Star Platinum instant yeast

10 grams of extra virgin olive oil

12 grams of coarse sea salt

1 / 4-1 / 2 cups of pizza sauce * see note

6-10 basil leaves

2 cups mozzarella with whole milk, freshly chopped

Instructions

To make pizza dough

Add the flour to a large bowl and make a large well in the middle.

Pour all the water into the well, leaving it intact.

Sprinkle the yeast over the water.

Shape the clay by hand and mix the yeast-water mixture, slowly add the flour to the wet mix and form a thick paste (think of a thick pancake batter).

Slowly start rolling a little powder off the walls of the well until you have a cloudy dough. Then add the olive oil and mix until it thickens.

Once all the oil is combined, add the salt and mix to make the mixture to be well combined.

Spread the dough out on a lightly floured board and knead, using slices of dough to form a ball of dough. The dough must be whole mixed and semi-smooth. Place the bowl on top of the dough, cover, and let sit for 20 minutes.

After 20 minutes, your mixture will look brighter and more relaxed.

Divide the dough into 2-3 equal parts and form smooth balls.

Put the dumplings on a tray and cover with plastic wrap. Or you can put it in a plastic container with a lid or zippered bags.

Refrigerate for at least 12 hours or a maximum of 2 days. (You can also freeze it for up to 2 weeks. Wrap it twice in plastic wrap and put it in a freezer container. Freezing dough in the refrigerator a night before.)

Heating things up

Place a rack in the bottom third of your oven. This is where the pizza stone is. When baking one pizza, it is recommended to use two.

Put another shelf on the top shelf and put another pizza stone there.

Set the oven to 550F.

Remove the dough out of the refrigerator 1 hour before baking.

Stretch the dough

With a mixture of 80% flour and 20% porridge, sprinkle the counter with a little "club flour" and place a ball of dough.

Using your fingertip, start in the middle of the dough and gently move the dough towards the top, leaving what is known as "cornicione" or the raised edge of the pizza. You push the air towards the top edge(from the center to the corner). This will inflate you and give you that airy crust.

Then fold the dough and place the side that you have already pressed closer.

Repeat the above process pressing forward until you reach the edge, leaving holes in all directions.

Turn and continue to push the dough slightly forward and out, but try not to knead it thinly in the middle. Once the center is large enough to fit the handles, gently roll the dough out, leaving the center alone and working toward the edges without touching the side.

If the dough becomes sticky, dip two fingers into your flour and drizzle lightly. You do not want to rotate the flour dough; otherwise, it will be difficult. If you have a hole, that's fine.

Just put the mixture back on the counter and hook the hole.

Bake a Pizza

Sprinkle the pizza dough with club flour. You will have to get your pizza out. Put a stretched pizza dough.

Gently spoon with a little sauce, add the basil leaves and mozzarella. Shake the bark. If the mixture slips, it's a good idea to press it inside a pizza stone. If it doesn't roll, gently lift the sides and add a little more flour under the bench.

Work quickly, open the oven door and place the top of the pizza dough near the back stone.

 Pull the pizza crust toward you, letting the pizza drop inside the stone.

Close the door quickly.

Bake the pizza for 6-7 minutes, making it half-cooked using the pizza dough

To Serve

Take the pizza from the oven and put it in a pizza pan or on a large cutting board. To finish, drizzle with olive oil and freshly grated Romano pecorino.

Notes

Classic and straightforward fresh sauce

28 ounces whole peeled tomatoes (Leo uses Mutti Pomodoro)

One teaspoon of sea salt

Use a food mill to process tomatoes to get pulp and juice, Stir in the salt and use within two days or freeze for later use.

Brewer Yeast Recipes

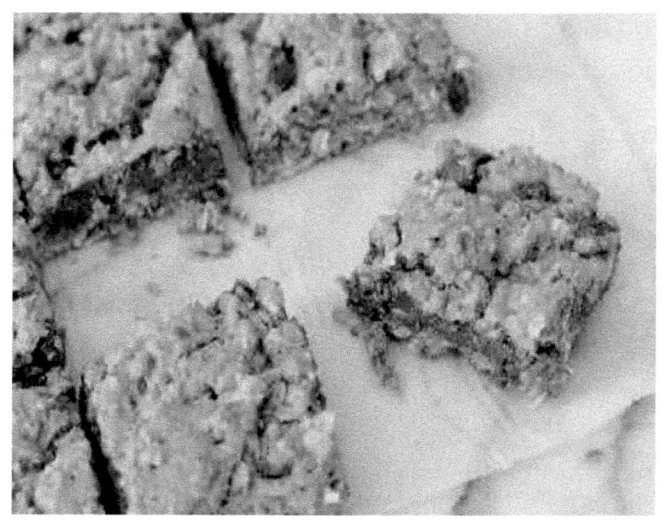

Total:

2 hours 30 min

preparation:

105 min Cook:

45 min

performance:

One loaf (for 6)

Nutritional guidelines (per meal)

104

calories

3g

grease

15g

carbohydrates 2

g

protein

Have you ever baked with a beer? Don't worry. This is very easy to do and requires no extra or strange steps. This loaf of bread is a beginner's bread.

Use only a mug of beer of your choice, and it tastes good after brewing.

It is suitable for sandwiches, snacks for soccer games, and to soak in a bowl of chili.

Ingredients

One package of active dry yeast

1/4 cup warm water

1 cup beer (room temperature) 1

tablespoon of cream cheese

1 spoon of sugar

1 1/2 teaspoons of salt 3

cups of bread flour

Put the ingredients together.

In a small bowl, mix water and yeast.

Stir until the yeast has dissolved.

Add beer, cream cheese, sugar, and salt to a larger container.

Pour in the yeast and stir.

Mix in 2 1/2 cups of flour.

Roll out on a floured board and beat the remaining half cup of flour or until the dough is smooth and smooth.

Place the dough in a greased pan and rotate the dough to grease the top.

Cover and leave to grow in a warm place for about 60 minutes, or until doubled.

Roll out the dough by hand.

Remove the flour dough and knead for about 1 minute.

Preheat oven to 375 F.

Roll the dough into one loaf of bread.

Put in a pan of butter.

Cover and let rise until doubled, about 30 minutes.

Roll out the dough by cutting three slices over the top with a sharp knife.

Place in the oven and bake for about 45 minutes or until golden brown.

Remove the bread and let it cool on a wire rack or dishcloth. Enjoy!

CONCLUSION

Hopefully, this book will motivate you to try and make your bread and pizza. There is no greater satisfaction than the smell of fresh bread baking. And when you bite a slice of fresh bread, it's pure heaven!

Remember, there's a lot of satisfaction in making and baking a loaf of bread. Even physical exercise alone, which includes kneading the dough, will release a lot of built-up stress, something that many people in the workplace feel from time to time. The pleasure of eating home-baked bread from the oven is a beautiful experience in itself. Try it and see what's going to happen. If your first attempt is not to your satisfaction, figure out what you might need to do differently and try again. The price of home-baked loaf ingredients is about 25 percent of what a loaf of supermarket bread would cost the financial cost of failure from time to time is rather negligible.

Always have it in mind that bread baking is a science and that you need to keep the ratio of liquid to dry ingredients in such a way that an edible loaf of bread is made.